# Detox and Heal

A mericans today are exposed to thousands of substances that didn't exist a hundred years ago. Insecticides, herbicides, fungicides, chemical fertilizers, preservatives, artificial colors, artificial flavors, chemical flavor enhancers, artificial sweeteners, automobile exhaust, electromagnetic fields, air pollution, radioactivity, water pollution, toxic materials in the home, alcoholism, cigarette smoke and drug use all place an unprecedented stress on the human body. The result, according to medical experts, is a weakening of the immune system and the creation of new illnesses.

Because we cannot escape the hazards of our environment, there is a growing public interest in foods, supplements and herbs that help strengthen the body and eliminate toxins. *Herbs for Detoxification* reviews the most widely used detoxifying herbs and detoxification therapies. It is an invaluable guide for strengthening the immune system, improving health and coping with the environmental stresses we all experience.

# About the Author

CJ Puotinen has studied with some of America's leading herbalists and is a member of the Herb Research Foundation, the American Herb Association and the Northeast Herbal Association. In addition to magazine and journal articles on health and medicinal herbs, she is the author of *Herbal Teas, Nature's Antiseptics: Tea Tree Oil and Grapefruit Seed Extract, Herbs to Help You Breathe Freely, Herbs to Improve Digestion, Herbs for the Heart, Herbs for Arthritis* and *Herbs for Men's Health,* all published by Keats Publishing, Inc.

A KEATS GOOD HERB GUIDE

MEDICINE
21 CENTURY

# HERBS FOR DETOXIFICATION

*Herbs to strengthen the immune system
and improve health by countering the
environmental toxins that surround us*

## CJ Puotinen

Keats Publishing, Inc. ✝ New Canaan, Connecticut

*Herbs for Detoxification* is intended solely for informational and educational purposes, and not as medical advice. Please consult a medical or health professional if you have questions about your health.

HERBS FOR DETOXIFICATION

Library of Congress Cataloging-in-Publication Data

Puotinen, CJ
   Herbs for detoxification / by CJ Puotinen.
     p.   cm.
   Includes bibliographical references and index.
   ISBN 0-87983-795-0
  1. Herb—Therapeutic use.  2. Environmentaly induced diseases—Alternative treatment.  I. Title.
RM666.H33P859  1997
615'.321  dc21                    97-4291
                                         CIP

Printed in the United States of America

Keats Good Health Guides are published by
Keats Publishing, Inc.
27 Pine Street (Box 876)
New Canaan, Connecticut 06840-0876

99  98  97      6  5  4  3  2  1

# Contents

# Contents

# Introduction

In an ideal world, all of us would enjoy perfect digestion and elimination. Whatever toxic materials we might ingest or absorb, our organs would neutralize and remove. Our systems would never be overwhelmed with material our bodies couldn't use, and we wouldn't store these wastes in our livers, fatty tissue and intestines.

But, alas, we do. Some of the toxins we absorb and retain come from our environment: cigarette smoke, air pollution and the countless chemicals we're exposed to; others we ingest in our food or the drugs we take. As we consume increasing amounts of processed and packaged foods containing artificial colors, flavors, chemical preservatives and residues of agricultural chemicals, our exposure to substances our bodies cannot use increases. The most debilitating exposures are to chemical weapons used in war, chemotherapy and radiation treatments used in medicine, prescription drugs with adverse side effects, environmental pollutants, industrial toxins used on the job, agricultural hazards such as chemical pesticides and, in our homes, outgassing carpets or insulation materials. However, even rancid fats, refined table salt, white sugar and refined white flour can be a burden.

What are the signs of toxic overload? They range from the symptoms of poisoning to less acute conditions such as fatigue, headaches, allergies, bad breath, an unpleasant body odor, hay fever, chronic bronchial or sinus congestion, dark circles under the eyes, skin breakouts, arthritis, memory failure, depression and lower backache to incomplete digestion, leaky gut syndrome, stomach bloat, gas, chronic constipation, chronic diarrhea, irritable bowel syndrome, ulcers, food sensitivities, a slow metabolism, weight gain and serious illnesses such as cancer. When not eliminated properly, wastes may not be expelled for days, weeks, months or years. Toxic materials that are re-absorbed into the body circulate in the bloodstream, interfere with the absorption of nutrients and provide a breeding ground for harmful bacteria and parasites.

However, toxic materials don't have to stay in the body. For millennia, people around the world have experimented with herbs, fasting and other techniques to accelerate the removal of toxins. By eliminating harmful material, detoxification therapies boost the immune system, improve digestion, eliminate the cause of many chronic conditions and stimulate good health, energy, optimism, mobility and stamina. The most ambitious detoxification programs have an impressive record of success in curing "incurable" illnesses, and even the simplest programs can improve the overall health of nearly everyone.

# What Is Detoxification?

Revising the popular sayings that you are what you eat or you are what you think, some nutritionists say, "You are what you don't eliminate." When your body holds onto unhealthy residues, it cannot operate at peak efficiency.

Your liver is one of your body's busiest organs, filtering the blood of bacterial contamination, secreting bile to break down cholesterol and removing residues of common prescription and over-the-counter drugs, caffeine, nicotine, carcinogens, insecticides and other chemicals. Your kidneys filter out toxins made water-soluble by the liver and excrete them in urine. Your intestines remove fat-soluble toxins excreted in bile as well as toxins from bowel bacteria; they complete digestion and collect solid waste for elimination. Your lungs remove gaseous wastes through exhalation. Your lymph system filters waste matter from inter- and intra-cellular fluid. Your skin eliminates fat-soluble toxins such as DDT and heavy metals such as lead through perspiration. Even your tongue is involved. Every hour of every day, your body works to remove what it doesn't need.

The natural health literature documents thousands of cures resulting from methods designed to speed and increase natural detoxification, including water fasting, juice fasting, eating only one food for several weeks or months, special diets, herbal teas, colon-cleansing procedures, high-temperature treatments such as saunas or sweat baths, massage therapy and salt baths.

## POPULAR HERBAL DETOX THERAPIES

Several herbal and nutritional detoxification therapies developed to treat cancer have proved effective for illnesses of every description. For example, the famous

Gerson therapy was designed as a cancer cure, but the Gerson Institute, which meticulously documents every case it accepts, has successfully treated heart disease, diabetes, rheumatoid arthritis, Alzheimer's disease and other illnesses with the same schedule of freshly pressed, raw organic juices and coffee enemas.

In the 1920s and 30s, Johanna Brandt, a native of South Africa, toured the world promoting her Grape Cure, the mono-diet that cured her of cancer. Brandt, who discovered her therapy by accident, influenced generations of natural healers by repeatedly proving, with her own case and hundreds of others, that a fruit or vegetable mono-diet can thoroughly cleanse the body, cure disease and nourish the patient, even during prolonged treatment. Brandt documented many cases like her own, in which a cancerous tumor grew on "normal" food but shrank and eventually disappeared if the person ate only grapes or other single fruits.

In Austria, Rudolf Breuss, a businessman and self-taught healer, theorized that cancer is fed by protein and that by going without protein for six weeks, one can starve the body's cancer cells. His theory became the Breuss Cancer Cure, a 42-day program of fresh, raw juices and herbal teas. Offered at clinics in Europe and North America, the Breuss fast has an impressive record of cures, not only of cancer but of many chronic and "incurable" illnesses.

Bernard Jensen, a leading figure in natural health circles, has treated thousands of patients with nutrition and high colonics, which are lengthy water rinses of the intestines. Jensen often relies on a mono-diet, such as raw apples, to begin the cleansing response. In one case, he had a patient drink only raw carrot juice for an entire year; this therapy cleared the man's body of debris, cured his chronic bowel disease and left him healthy and well-nourished. Jensen has inspired three generations of natural healers who have validated his teachings.

Harry Hoxsey, a self-taught herbalist, cured thousands of cancer patients using an herbal blend reportedly handed down from his great-grandfather. By the early 1950s, Hoxsey's Cancer Clinic in Dallas was the world's largest private cancer center, with branches in 17 states. Because of his popularity and success, Hoxsey was condemned, harassed and prosecuted by the orthodox medical establishment. However, two federal courts upheld the "therapeutic value" of his tonics and, in a landmark case against the American Medical Association, which Hoxsey won, that organization's president testified that Hoxsey's formulas cured some forms of cancer. Although Hoxsey was eventually forced to close his U.S. clinics, and although the American Medical Association, American Cancer Society and U.S. Food and Drug Administration condemn his name and therapy, Hoxsey's formulas live on. Andrew Weil, M.D., whose bestselling book *Spontaneous Healing* introduced many Americans to alternative medicine, uses a bloodroot paste like Hoxsey's for the topical treatment of skin cancers, and different versions of Hoxsey's herbal tonics are sold by herbalists around the country. These tonics contain plants known for their detoxifying properties, such as red clover blossom, buckthorn bark and burdock root.

Actor Jason Winters credits a tea made of red clover blossoms and chaparral leaf for his own cancer cure, and he became so enthused about this blend's healing properties that he launched his own tea company to share it with the world. Enthusiastic users spread the word that its daily use improved their skin, energy level, allergies, arthritis and other symptoms.

Essiac tea was developed in the 1920s by a Canadian nurse, Rene Caisse, who learned of an Ojibwa Indian tea from a patient it had cured of breast cancer years before. To the original blend of burdock root and slippery elm bark, Caisse added sheep sorrel and Turkey rhubarb root and named the result for herself: Essiac is Caisse spelled backward. For many years Caisse treated cancer patients in Canada with excellent results, and, like Harry Hoxsey, she repeatedly offered to participate in any clinical trial orthodox physicians might design. The offer was never accepted, although Canada's legislature came within three votes of authorizing such tests over the objections of its medical establishment.

In recent years, Essiac blends have been marketed by corporations that argue over its trademark and licensing while small herb companies quietly sell the ingredients that allow anyone to brew it at home. Every manufacturer and seller of Essiac tea has received reports of significant detoxification and health improvements in humans, pets and farm animals.

More recently, biophysicist Hulda Clark, Ph.D., caused a stir in holistic and orthodox circles with her *Cure for All Cancers*. Clark believes that cancer and other illnesses develop because of internal parasites, especially *Fasciolopis buskii*, which excrete waste material that stimulates abnormal human cell growth. The two ingredients in Clark's theory of disease are internal parasites and an impaired immune system. She blames exposure to pollutants such as propyl alcohol, benzene, xylene, toluene, methyl ethyl ketone and other solvents for the body's inability to identify and eliminate worms and microbes. Her therapy, which claims to cure not only every type of cancer but diabetes, high blood pressure, seizures, chronic fatigue syndrome, migraines, Alzheimer's disease, Parkinson's disease, multiple sclerosis, HIV/AIDS and other illnesses, depends on removing problem solvents from the patient's environment. In addition, she uses black walnut hull tincture, freshly ground cloves and powdered wormwood to destroy internal parasites in every phase of their development. Clark's claims remain controversial and her cures may be anecdotal, but the herbs she has selected have a long history of use for the elimination of parasites.

The approach taken by all of these therapies is that debilitating illnesses are systemic, not local; that they involve the entire body, not just a lung or a knee; and that by clearing the body of toxins that interfere with its ability to heal itself, a juice fast, mono-diet, herbal blend or series of high colonics boosts the immune system and removes the actual cause of disease.

# *Are You Ready for Cleansing?*

## THE IMPORTANCE OF pH TESTING

The body's acid-alkaline balance, which reveals its ability to adjust to the stresses imposed by juice fasting and herbal cleansing, can be measured by testing the pH (level of acidity or alkalinity) of blood, urine or saliva. Saliva and urine are the easiest to test; all it takes is a minute and the appropriate pH paper (see Resources).

Most Americans have acidic bodies that are brought into balance by eating alkaline-forming foods such as raw fruits and vegetables. Common sense suggests that if you eat acidic foods such as lemons and pineapple, your body will become more acidic, but not necessarily. Foods that are themselves acidic can cause an alkaline reaction in the body, and vice versa. This sounds confusing, but as you monitor your diet and your body's responses, the connection between food and pH will become more obvious.

According to Herman Aihara in *Acid & Alkaline,* the most acid-forming foods are rice bran, brown rice, wholewheat bread, fish, shellfish, egg yolks, oatmeal, chicken, barley, beef, pork, peanuts and cheese. The most powerful alkaline-forming food by far is seaweed, especially wakame, Irish moss and kelp (kombu).; Ginger root, kidney beans, shiitake mushrooms, spinach, cabbage, mustard greens, parsley, endive, carrots, strawberries, oranges and other fruits and vegetables are alkaline-forming.

The safest and most sensible way to approach detoxification is to spend several weeks preparing for it by eating foods that nourish and support the organs that will be most affected. See page 12 for precleanse or preparation-phase guidelines.

Richard Anderson, N.D., who developed the Clean-Me-Out program described in his book *Cleanse and Purify Thyself,* recommends the following tests to determine whether a person is ready for serious detoxification. If urine and saliva pH do not reflect ample alkaline reserves, he suggests continuing the pre-cleanse phase until they do.

*Please Note:* Juice fasting and herbal detoxification programs put a serious strain on the liver, heart and other organs. The following pH tests, which should be taken before you make dietary changes and again after two to four weeks of pre-cleanse preparation, will indicate your body's state of preparedness. If they show that you are not yet ready for serious cleansing, do not go on a fast or an ambitious herbal cleanse. Instead, continue the pre-cleanse diet for another week and test again. If you consistently test in the "too acid" or "too alkaline" range, consult a holistic health care professional who has experience with detoxification and cleansing programs.

For best results, use pH paper that indicates two-tenths increments on the pH scale between 5.5 (acidic) and 8.0 (alkaline). A pH of 7.0 is neutral. Wet the paper following label directions, and read it within 10 to 30 seconds. When the body has adequate alkaline reserves, a morning saliva test reads between 6.5 and 7.0; lower numbers indicate too much acidity in the system to proceed with cleansing. A pH reading of 6.0 or below may indicate a seriously depleted condition and any fast or herbal cleanse may be dangerous. A reading of 7.1 or higher may indicate stress or a mineral depletion that makes fasting unwise at this time. In case something has interfered with the reading, wait an hour and repeat the test. Saliva tests should be conducted after at least two hours without food, making early morning an ideal time.

Next, do the lemon test. Again, early morning is

best, but you can do this whenever you have gone for at least two hours without eating, or just after the saliva test. Squeeze the juice of half a lemon into a small amount of water, hold it in your mouth for as long as possible and swallow. Wait 60 seconds, then check your saliva's pH. Test again every 60 seconds for five minutes, for a total of six tests. If the pH consistently tests 8.0 or higher (very alkaline), it indicates good alkaline reserves, a reflection of overall good health. Readings between 7 and 8 show positive results, but Anderson suggests a third test (see below) before embarking on anything but the lightest of herbal cleanses. If your results are outside this range, fasting or serious cleansing programs should be postponed.

The third pH test examines urine. Because urine pH levels change daily, eating acid-forming foods for one day should acidify the next day's urine. However, in those who have mineral deficiencies, acid-forming foods create ammonia, making the urine alkaline. Take this test first thing in the morning after a day of eating "forbidden" foods, such as meat, poultry, fish, eggs, bread, pastry, fried food, canned food, etc.

A urine pH of 6.8 or above after a day on this acidifying diet suggests that the body has few or no alkaline minerals to draw upon. If this is your result, avoid strenuous exercise and focus on building the body's alkaline reserves by slowly increasing alkaline-forming foods (fresh, raw fruits and vegetables) and decreasing acid-forming foods. Anderson recommends doing this gradually unless you have a life-threatening illness, in which case time is of the essence and you should be under the care of an experienced healthcare professional. For all who test in this range, he prescribes ample quantities of carrot or carrot/celery/apple juice, mineral broths and an easily assimilated trace mineral supplement.

A urine pH between 6.1 and 6.7 suggests a mineral depletion that, while not dangerous, should be corrected before undertaking a fast or serious cleansing program. A urine pH between 5.7 and 6.0 is a passing mark, though by following the dietary guidelines below, you will continue to build alkaline reserves. A urine pH of 5.6 or below, which is very acidic, shows excellent reserves.

## WHO SHOULD NOT UNDERTAKE HERBAL DETOXIFICATION

While many women who were unable to conceive or carry a child to term have borne healthy children after detoxification therapy, it is not recommended during pregnancy. However, many of the guidelines suggested for the precleanse phase can be adopted during pregnancy with excellent results, especially the use of tonic root teas, raw fruit and vegetable juices, probiotic supplements such as acidophilus, the prebiotic foods that support beneficial bacteria, mineral-rich vegetable broths and dietary fiber. Consult an experienced healthcare professional for assistance in modifying the precleanse diet for pregnancy and breastfeeding.

Children of all ages have benefited from herbal detoxification therapy, but young children should be supervised by an experienced healthcare professional. The same is true for the elderly, the chronically ill and anyone who suffers from a serious disease, is addicted to drugs or alcohol or who has been exposed to dangerous chemicals, heavy metals or radioactive material.

# The Precleanse or Preparation Phase

For at least two to four weeks before beginning a detoxification program, follow these guidelines.

**Do eat** alkaline-forming foods, such as fresh fruits, raw and lightly steamed vegetables, salads made of four or more vegetables of different colors, raw fruit and vegetable juices, steamed potatoes, vegetable soups and sea vegetables or seaweeds. If you have been taking vitamins, minerals and other supplements, consider setting them aside during the precleanse phase as well as during detoxification. The foods and supplements recommended here are the most appropriate for this activity, and ample quantities of raw fruit and vegetable juices supply more essential vitamins, minerals, amino acids and other nutrients in a more easily assimilated form than most commercial supplements.

A diet based on raw foods and juices is so different from what most Americans are used to that you may need some culinary inspiration. If so, see the recommended "uncook" books in the Appendix. Learning how to prepare and enjoy foods that bring your pH into balance will make a significant difference to the success of your detoxification efforts and to your long-term good health.

If you are not familiar with ume plums, also called umeboshi plums, this Japanese delicacy deserves your attention. Made by layering ripe ume plums in sea salt and shiso leaves, the aged fruit is known as an effective blood cleanser, disinfectant and detoxification therapy. During epidemics, ume plums were used to prevent dysentery and typhoid, and Japanese physicians used them to treat victims of radiation poisoning after the atomic bombing of Hiroshima. Although ume plums and ume plum paste are widely sold in health food stores, the Japanese products are made with refined sea salt, a substance best avoided just before and during detoxification therapy. See the Appendix for an ume plum made in California with unrefined salt.

Because detoxification places a substantial burden on the body's mineral reserves, an easily assimilated mineral supplement (see Appendix) is recommended.

In most people, the diet described here is itself detoxifying. That is, it will probably produce at least some cleansing reactions. To help speed the removal of toxins from the body while reducing unpleasant symptoms, increase your fiber intake. Twice a day, add 1 teaspoon powdered psyllium husks (or a blend of powdered psyllium husk, apple pectin and/or other recommended fibers) to a glass of juice or water, stir or blend and drink quickly before it gels. Gradually increase your fiber consumption until you are taking 1 tablespoon. twice a day in juice, each serving fol-

lowed by a glass of water. It is important to drink
more water than usual, preferably two or more quarts
of plain drinking water per day. In addition, drink
herbal teas, especially those that are soothing and
relaxing, such as chamomile or peppermint, if you
feel stressed or anxious. For nutritional support, brew
tonic teas such as those on page 16. At night, just
after dinner or just before bed, take an acidophilus
supplement. For best results, do not take acidophilus
and supplemental fiber at the same time.

**Eat in small quantities** (a maximum of one serving twice per day, gradually reducing to one serving
every other day) cooked grains such as rice or corn,
and dishes made of dried beans or legumes. In place
of sugar, use small quantities of maple syrup or
honey and try to reduce the amount each day. Most
blackstrap molasses contains high concentrations of
pesticide residue, so look for organically grown molasses, which is a rich source of iron, an excellent
sweetener and an alkalizing food. In place of refined
table salt, use small quantities of unrefined, unpro-
cessed sea salt (see Appendix).

**Do not eat** acid-forming foods, which include any
and all breads or baked goods, canned or frozen
foods, pasteurized or bottled juice, dairy products,
eggs, meat, fish, poultry, nuts, raw or roasted seeds,
sugar, soy or tofu products, wheat flour products, distilled white vinegar, margarine, fried foods, foods
cooked in oil or packaged breakfast cereals, including
granola. Do not drink coffee, regular tea, soft drinks
or colas. Avoid tobacco products, second-hand
smoke, over-the-counter medications, recreational
drugs, beer, wine and distilled spirits. Avoid table
salt or any refined white sea salt.

If you are taking medicinal herbs, consider substituting teas or powders for alcohol tinctures, take the tinctures well-diluted in fresh juice or pour boiling water over the tincture in a teacup, which will cause most of the alcohol to evaporate. If you are taking prescription drugs, or if you have been treated in the past with drugs that have serious side effects, consult an experienced holistic physician or healthcare professional before planning a detoxification program.

# *Herbal Detox Teas*

It's easy to combine tonic herbs in flavorful tea blends suitable for drinking throughout the day not only during the precleanse phase but during more ambitious detoxification. Unlike some commercial "detox" or dieter's teas, the following do not contain laxative herbs or caffeine. Some of the ingredients, such as dandelion leaf or root, are mild diuretics that help rid the body of excess fluids without disrupting the body's balance of potassium and other minerals. These recipes are flexible and versatile. If you don't have an ingredient, simply leave it out or substitute something with a similar action.

These recipes are measured in parts, which can be teaspoons, tablespoons, cups or any unit of volume. Label and store each blend in a tightly sealed container away from heat and light.

ROOT TONIC TEA (decoction)
   *2 parts dandelion root* (Taraxacum officinale)
   *2 parts burdock root* (Arctium lappa)
   *1 part sarsaparilla root* (Smilax officinalis)

Blend ingredients. To brew 1 quart of tea, combine 2 Tbsp. tea with 4 cups water in covered pan. Optional: for a sweeter tea, add a pinch of dried stevia; for flavor, add 1 tsp. dried orange peel. Bring to a boil, reduce heat and simmer 10 to 15 minutes. Let stand 5 minutes before straining. Use between 1 and 2 tsp. tea blend per cup of water to brew larger or smaller quantities. Drink as desired.

GENTLE DETOX TEA (infusion)
   *2 parts red clover blossom* (Trifolium pratense)
   *2 parts dandelion leaf* (Taraxacum officinale)
   *2 parts stinging nettle leaf* (Urtica dioica)
   *2 parts cleavers or bedstraw* (Galium aparine)
   *1 part chaparral leaf* (Larrea tridentata)

Blend ingredients. To brew 1 quart of tea, pour 4 cups boiling water over 2 Tbs. tea. Optional: for a sweeter taste (the chaparral gives this tea a bitter, astringent flavor), add a pinch of stevia or 1 tsp. fresh-grated ginger. Cover and let stand 10 to 15 minutes before straining. Use between 1 and 2 tsp. tea blend per cup of water to brew larger or smaller quantities. Drink as desired. For notes on chaparral's safety, see page 66. If desired, substitute sage for chaparral leaf.

# Herbal Combinations to Avoid

Some products sold as detoxifying teas and diet aids have potentially serious side effects. For example, some popular diet teas and capsules contain stimulant herbs such as Ma huang or ephedra, caffeine-rich herbs such as kola nut or guarana, diuretic herbs such as juniper berry or buchu, disinfecting herbs such as uva ursi and laxative herbs such as cascara sagrada or senna leaf. All of these are useful and effective when used appropriately, but they don't belong in herbal tea blends sold to the public for weight loss or detoxification, especially with vague labels that encourage their frequent or daily consumption. Some of these herbs are ingredients in well-designed herbal cleansing products, in which case they are combined with other plants that help balance their action, but to rely on ephedra, caffeine and laxative or diuretic herbs to speed the metabolism, suppress the appetite and cause rapid weight loss is potentially dangerous. Just as ephedra created adverse publicity for herbal medicine when it was implicated in the deaths of young people who took overdoses seeking a legal "high," so have some dieter's teas been implicated in the deaths of young women. Constant overstimulation of the organs of elimination can create life-threatening imbalances of essential minerals, electrolytes and other nutrients, as well as dehydration.

Some herbal teas with "detox" in their names are more gentle and appropriate for daily use. But whether they come from the Ayurvedic practices of ancient India, European herbology, Chinese medicine or other traditions, these teas work best in combination with a diet based on fresh fruits and vegetables, gentle sources of dietary fiber and "green" foods.

Other combinations to avoid, although the consequences of violating these rules are less serious, are blends of fiber, herbs, clay, acidophilus and enzymes. After experimenting with several herbal detoxification therapies, I agree with Richard Anderson, who wrote that herbs which release mucoid matter from the intestines or which nourish and feed the intestines have the opposite effect of fiber and clay, which attract toxins, bacteria and debris. Fiber and clay work well together, holding released toxins in a single mass for evacuation, but any enzymes, herbs or friendly bacteria ingested with them will be trapped and never released to do their job. As Anderson explained, "These substances are excellent by themselves but ineffective when mixed together and taken all at once."

For best results, take clay and fiber together at least 90 minutes before or after taking herbs. Save acidophilus supplements for the end of the day. Digestive enzymes can be taken with meals, which should be scheduled at least one hour before and after these other supplements.

# Feed Your Friendly Bacteria

**B**efore, during and after the herbal detox therapy, take acidophilus and other "friendly" or beneficial bacteria. Why? If you're like most Americans, you've taken antibiotics, and that alone destroyed the beneficial bacteria you were born with. In addition, most of us eat a diet that starves our bacterial friends while rewarding their enemies. Add a little stress and anxiety, and no wonder we need help. Probiotics, the term used to describe beneficial bacteria, are now sold everywhere, even in supermarkets.

When shopping for probiotic supplements, check labels for not only *Lactobacillus acidophilus*, the most familiar name in beneficial bacteria, but such strains as *L. salivarius, L. rhamnosus, Bifidobacteria longum, B. bifidum, B. infantis* and *B. breve*. Bifidobacteria are native to humans and colonize in the digestive tract if properly fed. Both lactobacillus and bifidobacteria help control the potentially harmful bacteria *Candida albicans*, which, when it proliferates, causes systemic yeast infections or candidiasis. Some broad-spectrum bacterial supplements include the transient microorganisms *Bacillus laterosporus, B. subtilis, L. sporogenes* or *Streptococcus thermophilis,* all of which aid digestion, improve immune function and fight infection.

Now that you've got them, feed them. "Prebiotics" are foods that support the growth of probiotics without nourishing harmful bacteria. One of the latest buzz words in prebiotic supplements is FOS, an abbreviation for carbohydrates called fructo-oligo-saccharides. Natural sources of FOS carbohydrates include onions, asparagus, bananas, Jerusalem artichokes (the flour of this root vegetable is sold as a food supplement) and naturally fermented foods such as unheated, unpasteurized sauerkraut, kosher dill pickles, pressed vegetables and the Swiss whey concentrate Molkosan (see Appendix). Whey is a favorite food of beneficial bacteria, and Molkosan is unique for containing none of the milk solids that make whey products difficult for those with a lactose intolerance.

## HOW TO PRESS VEGETABLES

The easiest way to press vegetables is to use a Japanese pickle press (see Appendix), a plastic container with a screw plate that compresses the contents, but you can prepare pressed vegetables in a glass or ceramic bowl. Thinly slice, mince or grate green vegetables such as cabbage, endive or beet greens; grate or cut into paper-thin rounds or matchsticks vegetables such as onions, scallions, carrots, cucumber, red radish, celery or bell peppers. Knead and mix the vegetables with a sprinkling of unrefined sea salt (⅛ to ¼ teaspoon salt per cup of vegetables) until they begin to soften and shrink, or simply cut thin slices of any vegetable and sprinkle the layers with sea salt.

If using a pickle press, screw the pressing plate down to hold the vegetables firmly in place; if using a bowl, cover them with a plate weighted down with a clean, heavy brick or jar of water on top. During pressing, the vegetables combine with the sea salt, release their juice and form lactic acid, a vital nutrient for healthy intestinal flora. Note that this lactic acid is different from the waste product of the same name produced by muscles during vigorous exercise. Pressed salads have a complex, tangy taste and are easier to digest than the same vegetables served raw. They are nutritionally "dense," so that a small serving replaces larger servings of the same unpressed vegetables.

If brine does not cover the vegetables within a few hours, they need more crushing, a heavier weight or more salt. Press at room temperature. Cucumbers are ready within two hours, sliced carrots and other root vegetables within one to two days. Traditional sauerkraut and kosher dill pickles take more than a week to prepare in a ceramic crock. Any fermented vegetable or pickle made without direct heat or vinegar is an excellent prebiotic food.

Because the enemies of beneficial bacteria thrive on sugar, refined carbohydrates and other staples of the American diet, improved nutrition is as important as supplementation and the continued ingestion of prebiotic foods. Common responses to the dietary changes and supplements recommended here include the elimination of allergies, bloating, intestinal gas, irritable bowel syndrome, spastic colon, leaky gut syndrome, diverticulitis, yeast infections, chronic constipation, urinary tract infections and chronic fatigue syndrome. Because friendly intestinal bacteria strengthen the entire system, they are an important support factor in herbal detoxification.

# The Importance of Dietary Fiber

Dietary fiber, what remains of indigestible plant cell walls after food moves through the small intestine, makes stools soft and bulky, speeding their transit time through the large intestine. This dilutes the effects of any toxic or carcinogenic compounds in the intestine, causing them to be excreted quickly, and it helps remove or inhibit toxic bacteria in the colon. In addition, some forms of fiber attract toxins, absorbing and expelling them. Good colon health depends on fiber, and the lack of it has been linked to constipation, diverticulitis, diabetes, gastrointestinal disorders, heart disease, colon cancer and obesity.

Soluble fibers dissolve in water; insoluble or crude fibers do not. Both are necessary for optimum digestion. In fact, there are five types of fiber—cellulose, hemicellulose, pectin, gums and lignin—all of which enhance digestion and elimination.

The most popular source of supplemental fiber is powdered psyllium husk, sold by itself and as an ingredient in products such as Metamucil. For detoxification purposes, use plain psyllium husk powder, not products that contain sugar or flavoring agents. Also, for best results, use powdered psyllium husk, not seed.

Note that this effective bulking agent is a potential allergen. Some nurses who prepare daily doses in hospitals or nursing homes have inhaled enough of the powder to develop serious respiratory problems. Psyllium comes from *Plantago ovata,* a member of the plantain family (the garden weed, not the tropical green banana) and, as with any plant, too much of it can cause an adverse reaction. When measuring psyllium husk powder, keep your face averted or wear a pollen mask. Add a teaspoon or tablespoon of powder to a full glass of juice or water, stir briskly with a spoon, wire whisk or hand blender and swallow the liquid before it gels. Follow with another glass of water.

Sources of soluble fiber include whole fresh and dried fruit, dried peas, lentils, beans, barley, oats and seeds. Wheat bran is an insoluble fiber, and so is the roughage found in many vegetables and other whole grains. Vegetable gums, or hydrocolloids, are widely used in the food and beverage industry, where they help keep foods moist and act as a natural preservative. Among the 15 gums approved by the Food and Drug Administration for use in food are guar gum, derived from the seeds of the Indian cluster bean or guar plant and used as a thickening agent; carrageenan, a product of Asian seaweeds used as a jelling and thickening agent; cellulose gum or CMC, a chemically modified natural gum from wood pulp or cotton fiber; locust bean or carob bean gum, derived from the seeds and pods of carob and used as a thickening agent; and xanthan gum, produced by microbial fermentation for use as a thickening agent.

Fiber supplements that can be taken in capsules or used like powdered psyllium husk include glucomannan, a powdered root that absorbs up to 40 times its weight in liquids, giving a feeling of fullness that aids dieters and improves bowel function, guar gum (described above), which has similar properties, and pectin, the familiar jelling agent used in jams and jellies. Apple pectin is a mucilaginous fiber that absorbs cholesterol, prevents gallstones, reduces blood sugar imbalances and gently excretes lead, mercury and other toxins from the body. Pectin from apples, citrus and other fruits is sold as a food supplement in health food stores. Be sure to use this type rather than the sugared pectin sold for jam and jelly making.

Agar agar, a seaweed, is another source of soluble fiber, but it requires cooking for best results. Agar agar is popular as a mineral-rich vegetarian substitute for Jello.

Look for these ingredients in herbal blends or in their own containers at your health food store, and gradually add different types of fiber to your diet for improved elimination. Increase your consumption of water at the same time. For many Americans, the feeling of fullness that fiber produces is unfamiliar and uncomfortable, but it should become less so within a week or two. Adding too much fiber too quickly, especially wheat bran and other insoluble fibers, can produce gas and flatulence. If this unpleasant side effect occurs, take smaller quantities of supplemental fiber until your body adjusts and use carminative herbs such as chamomile as digestive teas. If you overwhelm a weak digestive system with too much fiber, or if your body is dehydrated, the result can be intestinal blockage.

Those who suffer from diverticulitis, Crohn's disease, irritable bowl syndrome, spastic colon and similar ailments must approach fiber with caution. In advanced cases, even the gentlest soluble fibers can cause problems. Although fiber is an important part of the cure for these illnesses, a depleted and damaged digestive tract must be healed before it can cope with whole foods. Fresh, raw juice diluted with an equal amount of water is probably the best initial therapy for these patients. See my book *Herbs for Improved Digestion* and consult a qualified health care professional for additional information.

# Detoxifying "Green" Foods

Cereal grasses (such as barley, wheat, kamut, rye and oat grass), alfalfa, aquatic algae (spirulina and chlorella), sea vegetables (kelp and other seaweeds), green herbs (alfalfa, parsley and chickweed) and other foods rich in chlorophyll are important in herbal detoxification programs. Much has been made of chlorophyll's similarity to hemoglobin, for both are blood: chlorophyll is the green lifeblood of plants, hemoglobin the red lifeblood of animals, and their molecular structure is almost identical. The hemoglobin molecule has iron at its center, while the chlorophyll molecule is built around magnesium, but in every other way, these two complex molecules match exactly. No doubt because of this affinity, chlorophyll is easily absorbed by the human body, where its healing properties can be dramatic.

Because chlorophyll helps to neutralize and remove toxins, green foods are important ingredients in herbal cleansing programs. The freshly pressed juice of wheat grass, barley grass and other cereal grains is available in many health food stores and can be prepared at home for daily consumption. Dehydrated cereal grass juices, chlorella, spirulina and other green foods are widely sold as food supplements. In addition to their detoxification properties, green foods help heal digestive disorders, combat fatigue and low energy levels, boost immunity and prevent deficiency diseases such as anemia.

# Clay and the Removal of Toxins

If you garden or spend time in the woods or along river banks, you know that clay is a dense, slippery mud. Most clays are rich in minerals such as silica, iron, calcium, potassium and magnesium, but their mineral content alone cannot explain their use as a healing agent for thousands of years. Some scientists have suggested that clay is alive, or that it has a negative electrical charge that attracts positively charged toxic material.

Powdered clay such as bentonite has such minute particles that its surface area is very large in proportion to its volume, allowing it to collect many times its weight in positively charged particles. Some clays are said to absorb and collect 40 times their weight in impurities. In *The Healing Clay,* Michael Abehsera described how contaminated water has been purified by clay, how in a famous French incident dogs that were poisoned survived after drinking clay water, how clay has prevented arsenic poisoning in people and how its external application has healed cuts, severe acne, infected wounds, eye injuries, fibrous tumors, serious burns and other conditions.

Clay comes in different colors, depending on its chemical composition and place of origin. One of the world's most famous clays is known as Cutler's earth, Luvos, aluminum silicate, colloidal white clay or balus. French green clay is a popular cosmetic item, and other clays are pink, red, yellow or gray.

The clay most useful in herbal detoxification programs is liquid or hydrated bentonite (montmorillonite) clay, but any powdered clay can be added to water and soaked overnight before using, with good results. In fact, even the thin clay water floating on the surface has impressive healing benefits. Adding thick hydrated clay to juice speeds cleansing dramatically.

*Please Note:* Michael Abehsera offers two appropriate cautions regarding the internal use of clay.

"Clay does not adapt itself to the presence of pharmaceutical medicines," he wrote. "Therefore, it is not advisable to combine its use with medical treatment." If you are taking prescription drugs that cannot be temporarily suspended, consult an experienced healthcare professional before embarking on an herbal detoxification program. "As clay is so powerful," Abehsera added, "it is advisable to precede clay treatment with at least ten days of purifying teas and food in order to reduce the amount of harmful toxins in the body."

# Support for the Liver

O f all the organs in your body, your liver will be the most stressed and overworked during detoxification. In order to keep it strong, healthy and functioning well, here are four liver support therapies you can use during the pre-cleanse phase, during the herbal cleanse (when your liver will be stressed the most) and during the months that follow.

**Liver flush.** As Rosemary Gladstar explained in *The Science and Art of Herbology,* "This famous liver flush sounds weird, tastes good and has wonderful effects on the liver."

*¼ cup fresh squeezed lemon juice*
*¾ cup fresh squeezed orange juice*

*1 tablespoon olive oil*
*2 to 4 cloves raw garlic*

Blend in the blender until creamy and frothy. Drink at least once a day (morning preferred) or in the morning and evening. One-half hour after drinking, follow with a warm cup of herbal tea such as peppermint or chamomile.

**Kudzu.** The root of the kudzu vine (*Pueraria lobata* and other species) is an important tonic for the liver in all detoxification programs, but it has a special ability to interrupt and help repair damage caused by excessive alcohol consumption. Look for Pueraria in natural food stores or herb tea catalogs, where it is usually labeled by its Latin name, or for imported *kakkon* (kudzu root tea), which may contain ginger, licorice and cinnamon as well. Some natural food stores and Chinese pharmacies carry kudzu root tablets and tinctures under the names *ge-gen* or *ko-ken*. If you're using dried Pueraria or kudzu root, brew a decoction by simmering 1 to 2 tsp. dried herb per cup of water for 10 to 15 minutes in a covered pan; let stand a few minutes, strain and serve. For a superlative liver tonic tea, combine 1 tsp. each dried kudzu root and milk thistle seed per cup of water and simmer as above. If desired, sweeten with stevia or organically grown molasses, another liver tonic. Drink 2 to 4 cups daily.

**Milk thistle seed.** The large gray seeds of *Silybum marianum* enjoy an impressive reputation after nearly 50 years of European research, where pharmaceutical grade milk thistle seed extracts are made for hypodermic injection as well as oral consumption. The seeds strengthen and tone the liver, are mucilaginous and soothing to the entire system and promote the flow of bile to improve digestion.

In addition to stimulating liver regeneration in cases of mushroom poisoning, liver disease and alcohol abuse, milk thistle seed is one of the most powerful yet gentle herbs for detoxification. It protects against common airborne pollutants distributed by the smoke of burning wood, tobacco, coal, oil and many commercially prepared incense products. In addition, the seed protects against X rays and the side effects of radiation therapy.

Milk thistle seed can be ground and added to food (1 teaspoon or more per meal) or brewed as a tea (see above), but it is usually taken as a tincture (¼ teaspoon or more daily, as needed) or in capsules (1 capsule 3 or 4 times daily). Like many herbs, milk thistle seed has a gradual influence and a course of treatment lasting at least three months is recommended.

**Castor oil packs.** The castor oil pack is a type of fomentation or hot compress that uses pharmaceutical grade castor oil, which can be purchased in drugstores and health food stores. Many herbalists, naturopaths and other holistic health professionals use castor oil packs as a specific therapy for the liver. The procedure is simple, and though it's time-consuming, it's relaxing. More important, castor oil packs help strengthen and heal not only the liver but other systems as well.

Select a piece of wool or cotton flannel two to eight layers thick, measuring 10 by 14 inches or larger when folded; saturate with castor oil. Place the cloth on the abdomen, especially over the liver area, cover with a plastic bag to keep things tidy (it helps to lie on a large towel while doing this) and top with a heating pad or hot water bottle. Lie still and let the pack heat up and stay hot for an hour. Wipe off the residue and place the oil-saturated pack in a zip-lock bag for storage. The saturated flannel can be reused for months.

Castor oil packs have been shown in clinical work to improve elimination in the gastrointestinal and genitourinary tracts, stimulate peristalsis, maintain the mucous membrane lining, improve assimilation, balance acid secretion in the stomach, stimulate liver, pancreas and gall bladder secretions, improve the functioning of major organs, glands and systems, stimulate the nervous system, regulate metabolism, improve lymphatic circulation and draw acids and infections from the body.

To support the liver for detoxification, you may want to use this therapy every two or three days during the pre-cleanse phase, every day during the herbal cleanse, then every two or three days for a week following the cleanse. However, any schedule will produce good results, so "use as desired" is an appropriate instruction.

# Support for the Lymph System

One of the least appreciated parts of the body is the lymph system. Lymph is the clear fluid that contains lymphocytes (the immune system's T-cells and B-cells) and which circulates through lymph channels to filter waste and bacteria from the bloodstream. Lymph circulation improves with active exercise and deep diaphragmatic breathing. According to Robert Gray, author of *The Colon Health Handbook,* skin brushing is as effective as lymph massage in cleansing the lymph system, removing stagnant accumulations of old waste matter. Daily brushing with a dry vegetable fiber bath brush, starting at the soles of the feet and working up the legs and trunk to the heart, then moving from the palms of the hands up the arms, then across the back and the abdomen, helps eliminate lymph mucoid through the bowels. "When practiced daily for several months," Gray wrote, "skin brushing is very effective for improving body tone. Five minutes per day of skin brushing is easily worth 30 minutes of vigorous physical exercise in this respect."

Additional support for the lymph system comes from herbs. Devil's claw root (*Harpagophytum procumbens*), a South African herb widely used in Europe in the treatment of arthritis and rheumatism, is both a stimulant of the lymphatic system and a detoxifying herb. Devil's claw is sold in health food stores. Follow label directions.

Perhaps the best known lymph-toning herb is cleavers, also called galium or bedstraw. The Austrian herbalist Maria Treben wrote that cleavers tea rids the liver, kidney, pancreas and spleen of toxic wastes. She recommended drinking it daily to tone the lymph glands and improve lymphatic health. Cleavers can be combined with other herbs and should be made as an infusion. Pour 1 cup boiling water over 1 teaspoon dried herb or 1 tablespoon fresh (double these measurements for medicinal strength tea) and let stand, covered, 10 to 15 minutes.

Other herbs that support, stimulate or help cleanse the lymph system include bayberry bark, sage, sumac bark, wheatgrass, burdock root, dandelion, goldenseal, yellow dock root, stinging nettle and red clover.

# The Importance of Water

Water, which is vital to good health every day, takes on special importance during detoxification. Extra water helps the kidneys function well, dilutes toxins in the urinary tract and prevents intestinal blockages.

No discussion of water would be complete without a caution regarding American tap water. Concerns over water safety have made bottled spring water a growth industry along with home water filters and distillers. A detoxification program requires clean, pure water that is free of added chemicals, harmful bacteria and parasites. Some nutritionists argue that distilled water is the only appropriate liquid for drinking, tea making and cooking, especially during a cleansing therapy, but others agree that any water will do so long as it is free from contaminants such as industrial chemicals, parasites and harmful bacteria. If you decide to purchase bottled spring water, look for clear rather than opaque plastic bottles or have spring water delivered to your home in glass containers. Avoid using any water that has an ''off'' or plastic taste.

# Exercise and Oxygen

As you prepare for herbal detoxification, don't just change your diet. Change your exercise and breathing habits, too. If you lead a sedentary life, this is the time to begin walking at every opportunity, breathing deeply while you do so. Strenuous exercise isn't necessary; what's important is that you inhale plenty of fresh air. The deep, relaxed breathing taught in yoga, biofeedback and meditation classes oxygenates the entire body.

For more rapid and thorough oxygenation, some authorities recommend taking hydrogen peroxide internally. While hydrogen peroxide and similar products have an enthusiastic following, this approach remains controversial even in holistic health circles. Hydrogen peroxide can produce more rapid detoxification, but debate continues over its long-term effects, short-term side effects and effectiveness. None of the authorities cited here advocate the ingestion or injection of hydrogen peroxide during detoxification.

See the Appendix for information about the five rites, a series of simple movements that by themselves can have a detoxifying effect.

# *Schedule for Pre-cleanse (Preparation) Phase*

Adjust times for personal schedule, maintaining, as much as possible, the intervals indicated here.

**6:00 a.m.**   Liver flush (see pages 28–29).
Raw fruit or raw juice as desired.
Herbal tea as desired (all day).
Plain water as desired (all day, 2 quarts or more).
Dry skin brushing (see page 32).

**8:00 a.m.**   Juice with mineral supplement (see Appendix).

**10:00 a.m.**   Juice with 1 tsp. powdered psyllium

|  |  |
|---|---|
|  | husk or psyllium/apple pectin combination (gradually increase to 1 Tbsp. fiber). Follow with 1 glass water. |
| **12:00 noon** | Salad with Molkosan or pressed salad, raw or lightly steamed vegetables, vegetable soup, fruit, juice, 1 serving rice or millet cooked with umeboshi plum or kelp, other appropriate dishes. |
|  | Nutritional supplements, as appropriate (milk thistle seed for liver support, green foods, digestive enzymes, etc.) |
|  | Herbal tea as desired (tonic herbs recommended). |
| **3:00 p.m.** | Juice with psyllium/pectin, as above. 1 glass water. |
| **4:30 p.m.** | Juice with mineral supplement, as above. |
| **6:00 p.m.** | Pressed vegetables, 1 serving cooked beans or millet, baked or steamed potatoes, vegetable soup, other appropriate foods and supplements as desired. |

**Before bed:** Acidophilus/bifidus/beneficial bacteria supplement. Follow this schedule for at least two weeks; test pH before progressing to more intensive cleansing.

# Cleansing Reactions

During detoxification, the organs of elimination work overtime. As they excrete material that the body doesn't need, they produce symptoms known as cleansing reactions. When the reactions are sufficiently dramatic, they are called a healing crisis, a term derived from the health improvements that typically follow detoxification. Beata Bishop, who recounted her Gerson Therapy experience in *My Triumph Over Cancer*, and Dirk Benedict, who told the story of his macrobiotic cancer cure in *Confessions of a Kamikaze Cowboy*, described the phenomenon well.

Cleansing reactions can take place at any time, even during the pre-cleanse or preparation phase. Symptoms vary, but in most cases, the skin, kidneys and intestines eliminate unpleasant-smelling substances, like truly malodorous sweat, urine and fecal matter; the tongue grows a gray or white coat of thick, unpleasant-tasting fuzz; the breath smells awful; the skin may break out in acne, rashes or other eruptions; the pulse may race; and symptoms like headaches, weakness, dizziness, fatigue, insomnia, nausea, sinus congestion and the intensification of previously existing conditions are common. If you have ever gone on a plain water fast, you know that these symptoms arrive in a hurry; if you switch from the standard American diet to vegetarian food or eliminate wheat and dairy products or adopt macrobiotic fare or a raw food diet, they occur more gently and over a longer period of time, but they still take place.

In some cases, the cleansing reaction is caused or exacerbated by the rapid destruction of internal parasites, *Candida albicans* yeast cells or other pathogens. The waste products of these organisms are difficult for the body to deal with when they are alive; when billions suddenly die, their decomposing remains have to be disposed of as well.

Dramatic cleansing reactions, although some people swear by them, are not necessarily desirable, for in the case of serious illness or exposure to toxic chemicals, the liver and other organs of detoxification and elimination are overworked. In extreme cases, sudden detoxification can be fatal. People who are young, healthy, active, health-conscious, well-nourished and free from major toxins can embark on the most arduous cleansing programs with good results and few side effects, but for most of us, ambitious programs are best approached with caution and common sense. Severe cleansing reactions can be incapacitating and truly painful. It isn't necessary for most people to suffer in order to rid their bodies of stored toxins, and the unpleasant side effects of detoxification can be minimized, even in those who have seriously toxic conditions.

Effective and relatively painless detoxification programs are those that work slowly, over a period of months or years. They rely on dietary fiber, freshly prepared raw juices, herbs that support a gradual improvement in health, toxin-absorbing foods or supplements and a gradual but significant change of diet. Fruits and fruit juices speed cleansing reactions, while vegetables and vegetable juices slow them down. Cooked, pasteurized, bottled, baked, fried, refined or processed foods, especially foods like bread, meat, eggs and poultry, can stop them altogether.

Nutritionists who specialize in detoxification say that if going without a particular food creates unpleasant symptoms, you're better off without it, for your constant consumption of that food (wheat and dairy foods are common culprits) is both masking other problems and making them worse.

How can you make detoxification more pleasant?

One way is to make the change gradually, which slows the cleansing reaction. Instead of eating wheat five times a day, have it once and substitute non-wheat items for the rest. This will help you grow used to thinking of other foods when you crave wheat and prevent some of the symptoms that would otherwise discourage you from continuing your new diet. If you're trying to cut back on caffeine, substitute relaxing herbal teas such as chamomile for half the coffee you drink, add extra hot water to the coffee you do drink, stop drinking colas that contain caffeine and drink more water. If you're starting the precleanse phase after years of fast food and cigarettes, a single day of fruits and vegetables can produce a splitting headache. Read the following strategies for reducing or eliminating cleansing reactions before making dietary changes.

When you're ready to try a more ambitious approach to cleansing, such as the herbal detoxification program that follows, be sure your body has the necessary reserves to support this plan. Use the pH testing described on pages 9–11, and spend at least two weeks preparing for detoxification by following the pre-cleanse diet described on pages 35–36. If that diet generates cleansing reactions, you can be sure that a more ambitious program will generate more sensational symptoms. Stay on the pre-cleanse diet until you are completely free of cleansing symptoms and your pH levels show healthy alkaline reserves. If you suffer from a serious illness, be sure to work with a qualified healthcare professional during every phase of detoxification.

To help your body eliminate toxins and reduce cleansing reaction symptoms at the same time, use any or all of the following strategies.

**Clay to the rescue.** Stir 1 Tbsp. liquid clay (see resources in the Appendix) into 8 oz. juice or use a blender and add 1 tsp. to 1 Tbsp. powdered clay to 8 oz. juice. Letting this mixture stand for a few minutes, then blending it again helps reduce lumps. Just before drinking it, add between 1 tsp. and 1 Tbsp. powdered psyllium husk and between 1 tsp. and 1 Tbsp. powdered apple pectin. Mix well. Drink this combination quickly, before it has a chance to gel. Follow with a tall glass of plain water. The clay and soluble fiber will absorb and eliminate toxins in the digestive tract.

**Slow the reaction.** Remember that fruit and fruit juices speed cleansing while vegetables and vegetable juices slow it. Drink freshly made, raw vegetable juice or bottled lactic acid vegetable juice (see Appendix). Other bottled or canned juices interrupt detoxification, so they are not recommended. If symptoms are severe, slow the cleansing process temporarily with a small serving of cooked rice or steamed potatoes.

**Treat nausea, headaches.** To reduce symptoms of nausea, drink a strongly brewed ginger root tea (use 2 tablespoons chopped fresh ginger per cup of boiling water and let stand for 5 to 10 minutes, or simmer 1 tablespoon powdered ginger per cup of water for 10 minutes in a covered pan) or take enough ginger in capsules to produce a warm, heartburn-like sensation at the back of the throat.

If you experience a headache, rub lavender or sandalwood massage oil into your temples or try the tofu-ginger poultice that has brought relief to many migraine headache sufferers. Drain 1 cup of chopped tofu until it is nearly dry and mix it with 2 to 3 tablespoons freshly grated ginger root. Spread the resulting paste ½-inch thick on a folded handkerchief or paper towel. Lie down and place the poultice across your forehead. Leave on for 20 to 30 minutes, then remove and rinse.

**Hyperthermia.** For centuries, the high temperatures of a sauna, steam bath or sweat lodge have brought relief from cleansing symptoms. Heat therapy is said to have a passive cardiovascular conditioning effect, relieve the pain of arthritis and rheumatism, improve blood circulation, improve the skin, reduce tension and flush impurities and toxins from the body. In the traditional Finnish sauna, a wood stove covered with rocks heats a wood-paneled room to about 200 degrees Fahrenheit. Water thrown onto the hot rocks causes a temporary increase in humidity and, with it, the sensation of increased temperature, but humidity drops rapidly as the walls absorb moisture. One time-honored way to take a sauna is to stay until you're thoroughly hot, then dive into a cold lake or roll in the snow and return for another cycle. That's one way to keep the circulation going! People who attend Native American sweat lodge ceremonies experience a similar sensation when they move between the hot, steam-filled tent and the cool outdoors. Saunas, sweat lodges, steam baths and hot water baths raise the body's core temperature in a mild and temporary fever that accelerates the elimination of toxins through perspiration.

Research in Finland, Japan and other countries suggests that fat stored near the skin's surface can be discharged in sweat and, with it, residues of substances that cannot be expelled through the lungs or kidneys, such as stored cadmium, mercury, lead, nickel, copper and other metals from chemical fertilizers, herbicides, insecticides, food processing and industrial chemicals. High-temperature sweat also discharges ammonia, uric acid and other waste products. Having grown up in a community that takes its saunas seriously, I agree with Finns who travel the world sorely missing this ritual: if you're used to a weekly sauna, you never feel clean without it.

Hyperthermia is not recommended for those with heart disease, circulatory problems, adrenal suppression, systemic lupus erythemotosus, hemophilia, multiple sclerosis or silicon breast implants. As this therapy raises the body's temperature, it is not recommended during pregnancy.

**Intestinal cleansing.** Enemas and high colonics clear the colon of toxins and reduce or eliminate the symptoms of cleansing while enhancing and speeding the process. In these procedures, water is applied rectally to rinse the intestines.

For an enema, which uses a small amount of water, such as one to two quarts at a time, the person takes in the fluid and holds it as long as possible before expelling it into the toilet along with intestinal debris. Inverted postures, such as lying on a slant board, lying on one side and then the other or massaging the abdomen, all help distribute the retained fluid.

For a high colonic, a therapist administers large quantities of water in a slow stream, which causes waste material to be expelled at the same time. It goes without saying that anyone performing high colonics should sterilize equipment between clients, maintain a relaxing and comfortable setting, respect the privacy of clients and provide accurate information.

Special equipment is needed for high colonics. Home units called colema boards (see Appendix) provide similar results without the need for an attendant and can be purchased from some health food stores and clinics or by mail. Drugstores sell the equipment necessary for enemas. Whatever your choice for home use, buy the best quality products you can afford, keep everything scrupulously clean and follow instructions carefully.

Be sure to use filtered, bottled or distilled water for intestinal cleansing, not chlorinated tap water. Chlorine can destroy friendly lactobacteria residing in the colon.

Can detoxification be completed without enemas or high colonics? Of course. But whenever detoxification is taking place, the body will from time to time be overwhelmed and all the symptoms described as cleansing reactions seem to take place at once. The more ambitious the cleansing program, the more extreme the reaction. These intestinal cleansing procedures, as unpleasant as they may sound, offer so many benefits that most people who try them swear by them.

Don't enemas and high colonics ruin intestinal tone and make users dependent on them, the way strong laxatives do? No, say the experts, because this therapy's purpose is not to stimulate intestinal activity but rather to remove debris. As long as the injected fluid is slightly cooler than body temperature, it has a toning effect on intestinal muscles. Warmer water is not recommended because it has the opposite result. After a thorough rinsing of the colon, it may take several days to resume daily bowel movements, but this is normal; it doesn't mean that the intestines aren't working properly or that they can't function without a laxative or enema. They're simply empty.

The Gerson Therapy relies on strongly brewed coffee enemas, which are said to stimulate the liver and cleanse the intestines without causing a caffeine reaction. I know from experience that someone who isn't used to drinking coffee and who is able to retain the fluid for several minutes before expelling it can absorb enough caffeine to feel jittery for hours, but an occasional coffee enema can relieve the symptoms of rapid cleansing almost immediately. Coffee is not your only option. Any herbal tea can be used, or plain water, or plain water mixed with clay. According to Bernard Jensen, clay and coffee should not be used together as these substances counteract each other.

To further improve intestinal health and reduce unpleasant cleansing reactions, follow intestinal cleansing with a rectal implant. Ann Wigmore used wheatgrass juice for this purpose, explaining, "The implants work to purge the colon and liver and to nourish the body via absorption in the colon." For a wheatgrass implant, fill a sterilized infant enema syringe or 3-ounce rubber adult ear syringe with freshly pressed wheatgrass juice, or use thawed frozen juice from the health food store, mix powdered wheatgrass juice with water or substitute barleygrass or other "green" juices or powders. This small amount of fluid can be retained by most people for several hours, but even a few minutes can be beneficial. Nutrients delivered in this way have not been altered by the digestive process and so have a different effect than they would have if swallowed.

In *Acidophilus and Colon Health,* David Webster gave detailed instructions for implanting bifidus bacteria, which may be the fastest way to establish a healthy colony of beneficial bacteria in those whose population has been disrupted by antibiotics or other causes. This procedure is best done at the end of a detoxification program, when the bacteria will be left undisturbed in a clean, hospitable environment.

To prepare for a bacterial implant, Webster recommended cleansing the colon with an acidic whey wash, mixing 2 Tbsp. powdered whey (if using Molkosan, use 1 Tbsp. as it is more concentrated) with 1 quart water for use as an enema. Retain the liquid as long as possible before expelling it, and massage the intestines to improve its distribution while lying on the left and then right sides. This procedure, which can be repeated for two or three days, creates a more favorable environment for beneficial bacteria.

Immediately after the final cleansing, mix 1 Tbsp. whey in 2 cups (1 pint) distilled or filtered water. Add enough of a bifidus supplement to supply 50 billion live bifidobacteria, which is sometimes called "human" acidophilus (see Appendix and compare product labels).

Rectally inject as much of this mixture as possible and try to retain it overnight or for as long as possible. In some people, an adjustment period lasting several days follows the implant and produces temporary bloating or flatulence, symptoms that usually disappear within a week. Strong chamomile, ginger, peppermint and other carminative herb teas help reduce the reaction.

**Herbal Melange.** Practically unknown in the U.S., Herbal Melange (see Appendix) is a mud-brown liquid peat that contains inorganic and organic materials, trace elements of over 380 healing herbs, minerals, vitamins and biologically active substances. One teaspoon taken 2 or 3 times daily in juice or water has been shown to cleanse and purify the digestive tract, stimulate digestion, bind gases and intestinal impurities, preventing their entrance into the bloodstream, lower the body's alcohol level, reduce serum cholesterol, create an environment hostile to harmful bacteria and parasites, detoxify the entire gastrointestinal system, including after X rays, and promote restful sleep.

Extensively tested by the Hygienic Institute of the Austrian University in Vienna and by the Moor Research Institute in Austria, Herbal Melange contains no drugs and there is no danger of overdosing. Prolonged use is beneficial and recommended since it protects against gastrointestinal disorders and supports the liver, kidneys, gallbladder and pancreas. Herbal Melange is recommended for people of all ages, including children and pregnant women.

Before, during and after herbal detoxification, Herbal Melange can be used to supplement the diet. During detoxification therapy, it can be added to the water used in enemas or high colonics to reduce cleansing reactions without interrupting the cleansing process.

**Natur-Earth.** Until recently, human beings ingested soil-based organisms (SBOs) every day. These beneficial bacteria live on freshly harvested vegetables, especially root crops, and some researchers believe that without them, our health has deteriorated.

In the late 1980s, scientist Peter Smith discovered large colonies of SBOs while hiking in a foreign country. Intrigued, he carried samples home. The result of his research is an unusual strain of bacteria now sold as the food supplement Natur-Earth. According to Stanley Weinberger in *Candida Albicans: The Quiet Epidemic,* Natur-Earth has helped cure many serious illnesses and chronic disorders, including candidiasis. In addition, its users report immunity from colds and flu, improved digestion, the elimination of constipation, improved metabolism, increased energy levels, resistance to infections, enhanced memory, and a long list of additional benefits. Natur-Earth is sold in capsules and has many applications in common with Herbal Melange, above. See Appendix for resources.

**Amino acids.** Ornithine and arginine, amino acids sold as dietary supplements, absorb and neutralize the ammonia produced by an acidic system, internal parasites or detoxification therapy. If you feel restless, uncomfortable, nervous or anxious, consider taking up to six 500-mg ornithine capsules at night, experimenting with the dose until you sleep comfortably through the night. Arginine, which promotes alertness rather than sleep, can be taken in the morning if needed, up to two capsules daily. After detoxification, cleansing reactions should disappear and the supplements can be discontinued.

**Relaxing herbs.** The relaxing nervines valerian root, skullcap, passionflower, chamomile and kava kava are widely sold as calming agents. In teas, capsules and tinctures, they help reduce cramping, tension, stress and anxiety. Take as needed.

**Tongue scraping.** Use a tongue scraper (see Appendix) to remove the unpleasant, furry coating from your tongue. No amount of toothpaste, brushing or mouthwash can accomplish what a single scraping does. Even when you aren't following the programs outlined here, this Ayurvedic preventive dentistry tool reduces plaque buildup on the teeth, removes toxins and helps eliminate bad breath.

In addition, hold 3 percent hydrogen peroxide (the strength sold in supermarkets as a topical disinfectant) in your mouth for as long as possible. When it threatens to fizz out, coat a damp toothbrush with baking soda and brush your teeth. The combination of hydrogen peroxide and baking soda will leave your mouth feeling clean and fresh. Repeat often. Herbal mouthwashes containing tea tree oil, grapefruit seed extract, bloodroot, echinacea and other disinfecting ingredients reduce the growth of unpleasant bacteria in the mouth.

**Nasal rinsing.** Sinus congestion is a common cleansing reaction. To relieve it, use a Neti Pot (see Appendix) or nasal douche apparatus from your local pharmacy to rinse the sinuses with a lukewarm solution of sea salt and water or salt dissolved in a strained herbal tea (chamomile and comfrey are soothing for this purpose) at about sea water strength. Repeat as needed.

**Exercise.** Exercise moderately. Fresh air and deep breathing are important now, but an ambitious detoxification program is no time to embark on unusually long hikes, jog at a fast pace or do hard physical work. Yoga and stretching exercises, especially inverted postures, are beneficial. An easy way to invert your body is on a slant board (see Appendix). By turning your body at least partly upside down, you relieve pressure on internal organs, stimulate digestion and elimination and increase the flow of blood to the head, all of which will help relieve unpleasant symptoms while supporting detoxification.

**Hydrotherapy.** Dissolve 4 to 6 pounds of Epsom salts in hot water in your bathtub, then fill the tub with comfortably warm or hot water. Immerse your body as completely as possible, add more water as needed to keep the bath warm and stay in the tub as long as possible, at least 15 to 20 minutes. Epsom salt baths help pull toxins from the skin. If desired, combine Epsom salts with baking soda, salt and/or the laundry product borax, as all have similar effects.

If time permits, dry yourself off and rest in a warm bed for half an hour.

**Aromatherapy.** Prepare a massage oil (see page 63) with lavender and sandalwood oils, or any favorite essential oils. Lavender and sandalwood are gentle to the skin, pleasant smelling, deodorizing and calming. Apply this oil all over your body as often as desired. Wipe off the excess with a damp washcloth or towel.

For a pleasant detoxifying bath experience, place a mat or towel in your empty tub. Add a generous quantity of massage oil to a handful of finely ground salt and mix well. Massage this fragrant, slightly abrasive mixture into your feet, legs, knees, abdomen, hips, arms, shoulders, elbows and back. Fill the tub with warm water and additional salt, relax, then rinse off. Be sure to use a mat or towel to stand on; the oil you massage into your skin will make the tub slippery.

**Castor oil packs.** Use this therapy (see pages 30–31) as often as desired to support the liver and other organs, gently stimulate intestinal activity, boost the immune system and help you relax.

**Reflexology.** Refer to a foot reflexology chart and massage the feet, pressing pressure points associated with the liver, intestines and other organs of digestion and elimination. Or, because all of these points are likely to feel sore and sensitive, simply massage the feet and focus on any point that feels tender.

**Skin brushing.** Using a dry vegetable fiber brush from a bath supply or health food store, gently and vigorously brush from the toes up your feet and legs, then from your fingers up your arms and shoulders, always moving toward the heart. Skin brushing stimulates the lymph system and helps remove toxins.

**Drink more water.** Dehydration is the enemy of healthy detoxification. In addition to tea and fresh juice, try to drink between a quart and a gallon of clean, pure water daily. Drink additional water whenever you exercise, take a sauna or steam bath, walk or work outdoors in hot weather or experience cleansing reactions. During detoxification therapy, drink water slowly; its rapid consumption can trigger headaches or discomfort.

# Detoxification Programs

You have spent at least two weeks changing your diet as described in the pre-cleanse phase, and your pH tests show that you are ready for a more ambitious detoxification program. Before considering the following options, review your calendar. The programs described here work best in a relaxed, familiar setting with a flexible schedule—not during hectic holidays, work deadlines or travel.

**Mono-diet.** You can embark on a mono-diet, eating

only one food (raw apples, for example, or carrot juice or raw grapes) for several days. This approach is guaranteed to produce cleansing reactions, so be prepared to deal with unpleasant symptoms. In most people who have completed the pre-cleanse phase and whose pH tests show good alkaline reserves, these reactions pass within two to three days and the result is dramatically improved health.

**One-day-a-week fast.** In *Inner Cleansing,* Carlson Wade described several one-day juice fasts, such as a lemon juice fast (the juice of six to eight lemons in a gallon of water, sipped throughout the day, with additional water as desired) repeated once a week to relieve allergies. In *Tissue Cleansing through Bowel Management,* Bernard Jensen recommended consuming nothing but fresh juice or raw fruit one day per week while resting, which he considered as important as going without food. Because the usual diet is resumed the next day, interrupting detoxification, this program minimizes cleansing reactions.

**Four-day (or longer) fruit or juice fast.** A four-day mono-diet juice fast, such as Jensen's watermelon flush (nothing but watermelon and water for four to five days) or Johanna Brandt's grape cure (nothing but grapes and grape juice) stimulates the kidneys and colon to eliminate toxins. In his classic book *Live Food Juices,* published in 1957 and now in its 39th printing, H.E. Kirschner, M.D., presented fascinating photographs and case studies of children, adults and even family dogs who were cured of fatal illnesses by raw carrot juice and other raw fruit and vegetable juices. Cleansing reactions are inevitable on this highly effective, therapeutic program.

**Herbal detoxification.** The most ambitious of the cleansing programs reviewed here, herbal detoxification begins as a modified juice fast, in which breakfast is replaced with fresh raw juice, while lunch and dinner are as described in the pre-cleanse phase. In addition to the herbal teas described on page 16, this program uses the following herbs in capsules. Check product labels for similar formulas, or make your own (see pages 62–63 for information on filling capsules). Do not use cleansing products that combine clay and fiber with herbs or acidophilus, as these key ingredients should be taken separately.

## Formula I

   *3 parts plantain leaf* (Plantago spp.)
   *2 parts barberry bark* (Berberis vulgaris), *Oregon grape root* (Berberis aquifolium) *or goldenseal root* (Hydrastis canadensis)
   *1 part myrrh* (Commiphora myrrha)
   *1 part Turkey rhubarb root* (Rheum palmatum)
   *1 part cascara sagrada bark* (Rhamnus purshiana)

## Formula II

   *3 parts dandelion leaf or root* (Taraxacum officinale)
   *2 parts cleavers or bedstraw* (Galium aparine)
   *2 parts ginger root* (Zingiber officinale)
   *1 part red raspberry leaf* (Rubus idaeus)
   *1 part fennel seed* (Foeniculum vulgare)

## Formula III

   *3 parts alfalfa* (Medicago sativa)
   *2 parts stinging nettle* (Urtica dioica)

    *2 parts slippery elm bark* (Ulmus fulva)
      *or marshmallow root* (Althea officinalis)
    *2 parts dandelion leaf or root* (Taraxacum officinale)
    *2 parts kelp* (Alaria esculenta)
    *1 part yellow dock root* (Rumex crispus)

Take any or all of these formulas in capsules with juice
or water between meals and at least 90 minutes before or
after taking supplemental fiber and clay; see suggested
dosages below. These herbs help loosen and release im-
pacted mucoid matter from the intestines, speeding the
cleansing process, while they nourish the blood, intestines,
lymph system and organs of detoxification.

Before beginning this program, follow the pre-cleanse
diet for at least two weeks and test your pH levels as
described on pages 9–11.

## SCHEDULE FOR HERBAL DETOXIFICATION

**6:00 a.m.**      Dry skin brushing (see page 32).

                  8 or more oz. juice with 1 Tbsp. fiber
                  (powdered psyllium husk, apple
                  pectin, etc.), 1 Tbsp. powdered
                  clay or thick liquid clay and 1
                  Tbsp. Herbal Melange. Blend well
                  in blender. Follow with large glass
                  of water.

**6:30 a.m.**      Herbal tea as desired (brew 1 quart
                  for drinking throughout the day,
                  see recipes on page 16).

                  Plain water as desired (all day).

                  Juice with mineral supplement (see

|  | Appendix) and 2 Tbsp. aloe vera juice or gel. |
|---|---|
| **7:30 a.m.** | Herbs: 2 capsules each Formulas I, II and II (or any combination of these or similar herbs), plus 2 capsules milk thistle seed or 1 tsp. tincture. |
| **10:00 a.m.** | Fiber/clay juice shake, as above. |
| **12:00 noon** | Lunch and supplements as in pre-cleanse diet. |
| **2:00 p.m.** | Herbs, as above. |
| **3:30 p.m.** | Fiber/clay juice shake, as above. |
| **6:00 p.m.** | Dinner and supplements as in pre-cleanse diet. |
| **7:00 p.m.** | Herbs, as above. |
| **8:00 p.m.** | Juice with mineral supplement and 2 Tbsp. aloe vera juice or gel. |
| **8:30 p.m.** | Fiber/clay shake, as above. |
| **10:00 p.m.** | Acidophilus/bifidus/beneficial bacteria supplement. |

For more ambitious cleansing, but only if your pH tests show good results, replace lunch with juice and herbal teas, then dinner as well. By separating clay and fiber from the herbs and acidophilus capsules, this schedule supports thorough and intensive detoxification, especially when juice replaces all solid food. The severity of cleansing reactions depends on the level undertaken and your physical condition. Use any and all of the suggestions on pages 40–41 to reduce unpleasant side effects. Within a few days of beginning this program, you will pass hard, rubbery mucoid matter from the intestines, an indication of deep level detoxification. These mucoid evacuations can be several feet long and weigh several pounds. For graphic color photos of what to expect, see Bernard Jensen's *Tissue Cleansing through Bowel Management* or write to Arise & Shine (see Appendix) for an illustrated flyer. Some people on the programs developed by Bernard Jensen and Richard Anderson have passed as much as 15 pounds of solid mucoid material, embedded wastes that laxative herbs, water fasting, fiber supplements taken alone and combination herb and fiber products do not dislodge.

## BREAKING YOUR FAST

Whenever you go for two or more days without solid food, or when you complete the program described above, returning to a normal diet requires logistical planning. The worst way to break a fast is to dive into large meals, especially items from the "don't eat" list. Instead, start slowly, focusing on fresh fruit and tiny servings of steamed vegetables and cooked grains. Your body needs time to adjust. Eat when hungry, don't overeat and continue to emphasize fresh, raw fruits and vegetables.

## ANTIPARASITE DETOXIFICATION

Parasites, once associated with foreign countries or the poor and unhygienic, are a fact of modern American life, *Giardia lamblia, Entamoeba histolytica,* cryptosporidium, *Trichomonas hominis,* flukes, tapeworms, pinworms, hookworms, threadworms and over a thousand other parasites can infect the human body and produce symptoms ranging from malnutrition and diarrhea to intestinal bloating, recurring indigestion, allergies, frequent colds or flu, candida yeast infections and exhaustion.

One popular antiparasite program is the combination developed by Hulda Clark (see page 6). Graduated doses of black walnut hull tincture, wormwood in capsules and ground cloves in capsules are taken on an 18-day schedule; the maximum daily doses are 2 teaspoons black walnut hull tincture, 7 wormwood capsules and 9 clove capsules, followed by a weekly maintenance dose.

You can combine anthelmintic or vermifuge (parasite killing) herbs with the pre-cleanse diet following the schedule Clark outlined in *The Cure for All Diseases,* or substitute the following in size 00 capsules. During the first week, take 2 wormwood capsules, 3 clove capsules (1 with each meal) and ½ teaspoon black walnut hull tincture daily. For best results, take these supplements before eating, on an empty stomach. During the second week, take 3 wormwood capsules, 9 clove capsules (3 with each meal), 1 teaspoon black walnut hull tincture and 3 grapefruit seed extract capsules (1 with each meal). Do not confuse grapefruit seed extract, a powerful vermifuge, with grapeseed extract, a popular supplement for the heart and circulation. During the third week, take 3 wormwood capsules, 9 clove capsules, 1 teaspoon black walnut hull tincture and 6 grapefruit seed extract capsules daily, at the end of which time your body should have eliminated any and all parasites in every stage of development. Every week or 10 days, repeat the second week's dosage for a single day as a maintenance program. Repeat the entire procedure every three to six months.

The pre-cleanse diet helps prevent parasites by eliminating their favorite foods. In addition, 4 garlic cloves blended in 1 cup water, strained and added to the water used in an enema or colonic irrigation helps eliminate intestinal worms.

Other approaches to parasite prevention were described by Hanna Kroeger in *Parasites: The Enemy Within*. Among her recipes: Combine 1 part cinnamon essential oil, 1 part tea tree oil and 1 part eucalyptus oil in 3 parts almond oil; take 4 drops once per day. Diatomaceous earth, used by gardeners as a snail and slug control, can be mixed with powdered psyllium husks (1 part diatomaceous earth to 1 part psyllium) and blended with juice or other liquids, 1 to 2 tablespoons per day, to combat intestinal worms. Foods that help repel intestinal parasites include cranberry juice, apple cider vinegar, pumpkin seeds, garlic and the white rind of pomegranates, while foods to avoid include raw or undercooked beef, pork, fish or poultry, sugars, refined carbohydrates, mountain water, wild water chestnuts and watercress, unwashed fruits and vegetables or produce washed in questionable water. To avoid this type of contamination, treat your kitchen wash water with liquid grapefruit seed extract (see package directions or my booklet *Nature's Antiseptics*).

## CANDIDIASIS DETOXIFICATION

If you are plagued, as many Americans are, with *Candida albicans* and the discomfort, yeast infections, thrush, ear infections, digestive disturbances, fatigue and allergic symptoms it causes, any of the preceding therapies should help reduce and control its overgrowth. Grapefruit seed extract is a specific for candidiasis. To be sure Candida doesn't return, take extra Molkosan and eat prebiotic foods (see page 20), replace fruit and fruit juices with vegetables and vegetable juices and drink pau d'arco tea throughout the day. The bifidus (human acidophilus) implant described on page 45 is especially effective in preventing this infection. Because antibiotics destroy beneficial bacteria, use these drugs only when necessary and reestablish friendly bacterial flora immediately after treatment.

# *Medicinal Herbs*

## HERBAL PREPARATIONS

There are many ways to take herbs: in teas, capsules, tablets, syrups, lozenges and tinctures, not to mention their external applications, like compresses, poultices and washes.

For best results, use herbs that were grown organically or wildcrafted, then dried at low temperature to maintain their flavor, color, essential oils and other properties. See the Appendix for herbal tea companies that specialize in high quality medicinal herbs.

If you are new to herbal medicine, remember that the recipes given here and in herbal reference books are flexible and forgiving. If you can't obtain an ingredient, find an appropriate substitute. Quantities are flexible, too. As you gain experience, refer to two or three different herbal references for information about each plant so that you have a clear understanding of its benefits, potential side effects and special requirements. Also, develop your own recipes.

Latin names are important because the same common name may be given to three or four different plants, or the same plant may be known in different parts of the world by different names, creating confusion. Latin names appear in recipes and when plants are listed individually.

**Teas.** To brew an *infusion* or steeped tea, which is usually made of fresh or dried leaves or blossoms, use 1 to 2 teaspoon dry herb or 1 to 2 tablespoon fresh herb per cup of water. Bring the water to a boil, pour it over the herbs, cover the teapot or container with a lid and let it stand undisturbed for 10 minutes. Strain and serve.

To brew a *decoction* or boiled tea, usually made from roots, bark or other hard, woody material, use the quantities given above and place the herbs and cold water in a stainless steel pan, cover and heat to the boiling point. Lower the heat, simmer the tea for 10 to 15 minutes, then remove from heat and let stand another 5 minutes before straining and serving.

Medicinal herbs can be sweetened with honey to improve their taste, or you can add flavors such as black cherry concentrate or fresh ginger or a pinch of stevia, the sweet herb widely used as a sugar substitute. Most herbalists recommend taking medicinal teas straight, with no added flavors or sweeteners.

**Tinctures.** To make a tincture, which is a concentrated alcohol extract, fill a glass jar ¼ to ⅓ full with fresh or dried herbs that you have cut or shredded into small pieces. Cover the herbs with 80-proof or higher proof vodka, rum, brandy, or grain alcohol, with a few inches of alcohol above the plant matter. Cover tightly and place in a warm location. Check the jar every day or two, shaking it briefly. As the dried herbs absorb the liquid, add more alcohol. Some recipes call for 1 part plant matter to 4 parts alcohol, but using less alcohol or more plant material results in a more concentrated, medicinal tincture. Let the tincture stand for three or four weeks before filtering. Some herbalists recommend straining and bottling tinctures at the full moon. There is no specific deadline; a tincture left for two months will be more potent than one left for two weeks. Strain the tincture through cheesecloth or muslin, pressing out as much liquid as possible before discarding the spent plant material. Alcohol tinctures have an indefinite shelf life. Stored in amber glass jars away from heat and light, they last for decades.

If you prefer not to use alcohol for the tinctures you will use during detoxification therapy, substitute vegetable glycerine or mix glycerine with alcohol. Glycerine does not dissolve all of the medicinal constituents that alcohol extracts, but it is widely used in tinctures, especially for children. Glycerine adds a sweet taste and syrupy texture to tinctures. Cider vinegar can be used to make no-alcohol tinctures, though their shelf life is shorter than glycerine or alcohol tinctures and vinegar does not dissolve as many substances within the herbs.

For an even more concentrated tincture, pour your filtered tincture into a jar containing new plant material and repeat the process. Small quantities of this "double strength" tincture will have a powerful medicinal effect.

There is much confusion about tincture dosage, a misunderstanding that herbalist Rosemary Gladstar attributes to the caution of small companies marketing tinctures in the 1960s. "The only similar products were homeopathic preparations," she explains, "and their doses are measured in drops. Herbal tinctures are entirely different, and they should be taken by the half-teaspoon, teaspoon or tablespoon, not by the drop." Anyone buying, making or taking herbal tinctures should know that disappointing results may not be caused by a tincture's herbal ingredients but rather by doses that are entirely too small. A few herbs should be taken in small amounts, but most of the tinctures mentioned here, such as milk thistle seed tincture, are safe and effective in larger doses. Tinctures can be taken straight or diluted in tea, water or fruit juice.

**Capsules.** Herbal capsules are widely sold and, if you need a special blend of herbs in capsules, some of the mail order herb companies blend and encapsulate custom orders for a nominal fee. Or you can put your own herbs into capsules. For best results, leave dried herbs whole or in large pieces until needed to preserve their essential oils and medicinal properties. Herbs should be stored away from heat and light in well-sealed glass containers for maximum shelf life.

When ready to use, grind them in a blender or spice grinder until they are powdered. To reduce exposure to herb dust, which can irritate nasal passages, wear a pollen mask. Two-part gelatin capsules, including vegetable gelatin capsules for vegetarians, are widely sold in health food stores and herb catalogs in sizes 0, 00 and 000. Many herbal companies sell mechanical capping devices that hold several capsules in place for faster and easier filling.

**Massage oils.** To make an effective massage oil for use during detoxification therapy, start with a carrier oil that's readily absorbed and has a neutral or pleasant fragrance, such as almond, apricot kernel, peach kernel, jojoba or a very light olive oil. These oils, which are sold in most health food stores, can be blended in any proportions.

The skin is an important organ all the time, but especially during detoxification, when it is kept busy eliminating debris through the pores and sweat glands.

The right essential oils turn simple massage oils into important support therapies for detoxification. Lavender, sandalwood and tea tree oil help cleanse the skin and relax the mind. Add several drops to an appropriate carrier oil and apply to feet, legs, arms, underarms, abdomen and back. Wipe off the excess with a damp washcloth or towel.

## SPECIAL DETOXIFICATION HERBS

The following herbs are widely used in detoxification programs, and you will see them listed as ingredients on many labels. Because space is limited, only the most important "detox" herbs are described individually.

**Aloe vera** (*Aloe vera*). While the bitter sap of this succulent's rind contains cathartic principles, giving it strong laxative properties, the inner gel or juice is a digestive tonic that soothes internal organs. Recent research has focused on the plant's high mucopolysachharide content; mucopolysaccharides are long-chain sugars and major components of other powerful immune-enhancing plants such as reishi, shiitake and maitake mushrooms, astragalus and ginseng.

Studies at the Linus Pauling Institute of Science and Medicine show that six ounces of aloe vera juice taken three times daily increased protein digestion and absorption, decreased bowel putrefaction, improved pH levels in the intestinal tract and demonstrated antibacterial, antifungal and antiyeast activity. Other research has shown that properly processed whole-leaf aloe vera juice destroys pathogenic bacteria, viruses, yeasts and parasites, helps break down and remove dead cells and toxic substances and reduces the side effects of radiation and chemotherapy. Add up to 1 or 2 ounces of aloe vera juice or gel to fruit or vegetable juices during the pre-cleanse phase as well as during detoxification therapy.

**Black walnut hull** (*Juglans nigra*). Black walnut hull powders and tinctures are popular anthelmintics: they help expel worms and other parasites from the body. In addition, this astringent herb is an effective treatment for diarrhea. Walnut hulls are green when they fall from the tree in autumn and turn black within a week. The green hulls of black walnut are prized for their superior benefits, making "green" black walnut hull tincture the preference of Hulda Clark and her followers, but black tincture has been used for centuries in people, pets and farm animals with good results.

**Burdock root** (*Arctium lappa*). An important herb for the liver, burdock root is a tonic, diuretic, demulcent herb. It is used to treat skin diseases, gout, kidney disease and bladder problems. Burdock root promotes kidney function and helps clear the blood of harmful acids. Research has shown that its seeds can lower blood sugar in rats, and in France the fresh root is prescribed for this purpose.

Burdock root is a common Japanese vegetable called *gobo*, sold in thousands of grocery stores and sushi bars and used in many herbal formulas. Years ago a single batch of burdock was contaminated with belladonna root, which contains the poisonous compound atropine. It happened only once, but some medical authorities still refer to burdock as toxic because of its presumed atropine levels. Burdock root does not contain atropine, and it has a long and enviable track record of safe consumption by large numbers of people over long periods of time.

**Cascara sagrada** (*Rhamnus purshiana*). Cascara is a powerful laxative, a purgative if taken in sufficient doses and a bitter tonic. It is one of the oldest and most reliable remedies for chronic constipation. Cascara is not habit-forming but is a good intestinal tonic and remedy for gallstones and liver complaints. It can be used in the cleansing phase of an herbal detoxification therapy to help speed waste material from the colon. Add a pinch of powdered cascara bark to tea or juice once or twice daily.

**Chaparral leaf** (*Larrea tridentata*). This bitter herb from the Pacific Southwest is a diuretic, tonic, astringent and anti-inflammatory that protects against intestinal parasites and some tumors. It has a sharp, creosote taste. One of the best herbal antibiotics, chaparral fights infections of the intestinal and urinary tracts and is effective in treating diarrhea caused by pathogens. Few herbs have chaparral's detoxifying properties, especially in combination with red clover.

Because of actions by the U.S. Food and Drug Administration in 1992, chaparral was labeled dangerous and pulled from many U.S. markets. After an extensive review of the herb's history by a panel of medical experts with specialties in gastroenterology and hepatitis, and after meeting with FDA officials, the Board of Trustees of the American Herbal Products Association voted in 1995 to resume the sale of chaparral. The board now recommends that anyone who has, or has had, a liver disease seek advice from a healthcare practitioner before using chaparral but that it be freely bought and sold.

**Cleavers** or **Bedstraw** (*Galium aparine* and other species). This diuretic, disinfecting, tonic, blood-cleansing herb is a specific for the lymph system, and it helps rid the liver, kidneys, pancreas and spleen of toxic wastes. It is widely used in European herbology.

**Cloves** (*Eugenia caryophyllus*). This familiar sweet spice is a stimulant, carminative, aromatic and vermifuge. When taken as part of a detoxification program, it helps relieve gassiness and flatulence, increase the action of other herbs and destroy internal parasites. For best results, use freshly ground cloves in capsules.

**Dandelion** (*Taraxacum officinale*). The familiar dandelion, from woody root to toothy leaf, is one of nature's most medicinal plants. Dandelion is a tonic herb for the liver and digestive tract, a blood cleanser and a diuretic. Eat its fresh leaves in salads and drink dandelion tea for improved liver function. Michael Tierra notes that serious cases of hepatitis have been cured with the use of dandelion tea in combination with dietary restrictions in as little as one week.

Brew the leaf as an infusion, the root as a decoction. Drink dandelion tea before meals or at any time during and preceding detoxification therapy.

**Garlic** (*Allium sativum*). Best known for its pungent culinary uses, garlic is one of the world's most researched medicinal herbs. Its regular use lowers cholesterol levels, protects against lead poisoning and toxins such as carbon tetrachloride, destroys a wide range of pathogenic bacteria, eliminates intestinal worms and boosts the immune system. Garlic's odor can be neutralized with green foods such as parsley or breath products taken in capsules; aged or deodorized garlic products reduce or eliminate the odor problem.

**Ginger root** (*Zingiber officinalis*). This familiar culinary spice is a stimulant, carminative herb that combats nausea, promotes circulation and relieves cramping. See page 41 for a ginger headache poultice.

**Grapefruit seed extract.** An extract of grapefruit or other citrus seeds and the fruit's connecting membranes, this powerful antiseptic has been shown to kill bacteria, viruses, fungi, yeasts, parasites and other pathogens on contact. Sold in health food stores under the brand name ProSeed, Citricidal and others, grapefruit seed extract is available in very bitter tasting drops or de-bittered powder capsules. Well-tolerated by people of all ages and having no known side effects when taken as recommended, grapefruit seed extract is effective in the treatment and prevention of traveler's diarrhea, infections of all types and chronic yeast infections. For more information, see my booklet *Nature's Antiseptics: Tea Tree Oil and Grapefruit Seed Extract.*

**Kelp and other sea vegetables.** Because they contain nearly every mineral and trace mineral necessary for human health, along with vitamins and amino acids, kelp (also called kombu) and other sea vegetables, such as nori (laver), agar agar, wakame, hijiki, arame and dulse, help prevent dietary deficiencies. The most alkalizing of foods, these seaweeds work quickly to correct the acid imbalances common to North Americans. In addition, they share an ability to pull stored toxins from the body. Seaweeds can be added to soups, stews and other foods or taken in capsules during the pre-cleanse phase as well as during and after detoxification therapy.

*Please Note:* Some people are sensitive or allergic to the iodine in sea vegetables, a reaction that can cause unsightly acne-like skin eruptions. If you experience this side effect, discontinue use and avoid products that contain iodine.

**Kudzu root** (*Pueraria lobata, P. pseudohirsuta*). Unappreciated in the American Southeast, where it has become a rampant weed, kudzu root is prized in Asia for its ability to reduce alcohol cravings, help reverse the damage caused by an overconsumption of alcohol and strengthen the liver. Its long history of medicinal use in China and Japan prompted U.S. researchers to experiment with it, using golden hamsters, a species notorious for its alcoholic capacity. When kudzu extract reduced the hamsters' cravings, it became famous overnight.

Kudzu tea, made from the whole root, is different from kudzu starch sold in health food stores as a thickening agent resembling cornstarch. Kudzu's flavonoids, which are believed to be the plant's active medicinal ingredients, increase blood flow, improve circulation and relax smooth muscle tissue. Brew as a decoction or look for Asian kudzu powders (see page 29).

**Lemon juice, lemon peel.** Used for centuries for health complaints of every description, lemon juice, lemon peel and pectin from lemons all help cleanse the body and speed the elimination of toxins use organically grown lemons whenever possible. Add lemon juice to water, tea or other liquids, and grated peel to any tea blend or add citrus pectin to any recipe calling for powdered psyllium husk or other fiber.

**Milk thistle** (*Silybum marianus*). Milk thistle seed is a powerful liver stimulant, tonic and healer. Important in the treatment of mushroom poisoning, hepatitis, alcoholic cirrhosis, drug damage and the damage caused by environmental toxins, milk thistle has been scientifically researched in Europe for over 45 years. In addition to improving the liver, milk thistle seed can be used for all gall bladder problems. Brew the seeds as an infusion, grind them and add them to food, or take capsules or tinctures. See page 30.

**Myrrh** (*Commiphora myrrha*). This Biblical resin has been used for thousands of years as a medicine and incense. Antiseptic, astringent, carminative and tonic in nature, it helps cleanse the body and supports detoxification. Myrrh's harsh, acrid taste can be unpleasant in teas or tinctures, so it is usually used in small quantities, combined with other herbs or taken in capsules.

**Pau d'arco** or **lapacho** (*Tabebuia avellanedae* and *T. impetiginosa*). Known in its native South America as *Ipe roxo,* pau d'arco contains biologically active substances that disrupt bacteria, viruses, parasites and fungi. The tree's inner back lining has potent anti-inflammatory, analgesic, antioxidant and immunotonic properties. Best known for its use in the treatment of Candida yeast infections, pau d'arco is an important herb for overall detoxification. Brew as a decoction.

**Red clover blossom, leaf** (*Trifolium pratense*). A mild stimulant, sedative, nutritive, antispasmodic and cleansing herb, red clover has a long history of use in detoxification. Well-tolerated by children, the elderly and people in fragile health, this herb is a specific for respiratory conditions. It combines well with other herbs and can be added to any tea blend. Brew as an infusion. To make an effective cleansing tea, combine up to 9 parts red clover blossom with 1 part chaparral. Use 1 tsp. of this blend per cup of boiling water and brew as an infusion. As you grow accustomed to the taste, which takes time, double or triple the amount of chaparral.

**Red raspberry leaf** (*Rubus idaeus*). Considered a specific for the female organs, red raspberry leaf does more than promote healthy pregnancies; its astringent, tonic properties gently support detoxification and help improve the entire system in people of all ages. Safe for children and nursing infants, it works well in combination with other herbs in teas, tinctures and capsules. Brew as an infusion.

**Sarsaparilla** (*Smilax officinalis*). Sarsaparilla's familiar root beer taste makes it a pleasant addition to herbal tea blends, and its diuretic, tonic, stimulant, demulcent and carminative properties make it an important digestive tonic. The famous American herbalist Jethro Kloss considered it an excellent antidote for poisons and found it useful in treating rheumatism, skin eruptions and ringworm. He recommended taking the tea (1 to 2 cups daily) or tincture (25 to 50 drops daily) for no more than two weeks out of every three. Michael Tierra advised combining sarsaparilla with sassafras and yellow dock as a spring tonic. According to him, a hot decoction (2 Tbsp. root simmered in 2 cups water) acts as a powerful agent to expel gas from the stomach and intestines.

**Senna** (*Cassia marilandica*). Also called American senna or locust plant, senna is a valuable laxative. It is recommended for indigestion, bad breath, a bad taste in the mouth and the treatment of intestinal parasites. Because senna by itself can cause cramps or spasms, it should be combined with aromatic, carminative herbs such as chamomile and ginger. As an anthelmintic (worm therapy) it works best in combination with other herbs in that category. To brew a decoction, bring 4 Tbsp. senna to a boil with 2 cups water and 1 tsp. powdered ginger, 1 Tbsp. fresh grated ginger and/or 1 tsp. fennel seed. Simmer over low heat, tightly covered, for 30 minutes; then remove from heat and let stand another 10 minutes. Drink 2 oz. (⅛ cup) at a time. Take this herb in small doses as it is a more powerful laxative than cascara sagrada. In most cases, it relieves constipation within six to eight hours. Senna is not recommended for use during pregnancy or by the elderly.

**Sheep sorrel** (*Rumex acetosella*). A wild perennial relative of garden sorrel, sheep sorrel is an ingredient in Essiac tea (see page 6). It is a blood tonic said to be beneficial to the heart, and it has been used to treat ulcers and kidney disorders.

**Slippery elm bark** (*Ulmus fulva*). A demulcent, nutritive, tonic and slightly diuretic herb with many traditional uses, slippery elm bark nourishes the digestive tract while it soothes the stomach and intestines. Because this herb is in short supply, many herbalists substitute marshmallow root, (*Althea officinalis*) which has similar properties. Both are rich sources of easily digested vegetable mucilage and can be added to fiber shakes containing powdered psyllium husk, pectin and other fiber.

**Stinging nettle** (*Urtica dioica*). Popular throughout Europe as a tonic herb and best known in the U.S. for its treatment of hay fever, stinging nettle is a blood cleansing, antiseptic herb. It combines well with other plants in teas, tinctures and capsules. Other than the sting caused by fresh nettle, this plant has no adverse side effects.

**Turkey rhubarb root** (*Rheum palmatum*). Native to China and Tibet but popularly known as Turkey rhubarb root, this relative of the domestic rhubarb is a powerful liver tonic, appetite stimulant, digestive aid and headache reliever. It is one of the four key ingredients of Essiac (see page 53).

**Wormwood** (*Artemisia absinthium*). A bitter herb, wormwood lives up to its name by helping rid the body of intestinal parasites. In addition, its antiseptic, antispasmodic, carminative and stimulant properties make it a tonic for the stomach and digestive tract. The distilled essential oil of wormwood, which is extremely concentrated, can be toxic and addictive: absinthe, a notorious liqueur that contains this essential oil, ruined some of the best minds in 19th century Europe. Wormwood tea and powdered wormwood capsules are considered safe in small quantities even for prolonged use; in concentrated doses, such as in the treatment of intestinal worms, wormwood can be taken for several weeks at a time.

**Yellow dock root** (*Rumex crispus*). The root of this nuisance weed is a buried treasure, one of the best known blood purifiers in herbal medicine. A gentle laxative, yellow dock root stimulates bile production and helps tone the liver. Like burdock root and dandelion root, yellow dock root improves digestion and the assimilation of nutrients, stimulates the elimination of toxins from the body and gradually restores normal body function.

# Bibliography

Abehsera, Michael. *The Healing Clay.* Secaucus, N.J.: Citadel Press, 1979.

Aihara, Herman. *Acid & Alkaline.* Oroville, Calif.: George Ohsawa Macrobiotic Foundation, 1986.

Anderson, Richard. *Cleanse and Purify Thyself: The Clean-Me-Out Program.* Tucson, Ariz.: Richard Anderson, 1988.

Baker, Mark A. *Colon Irrigation: A Forgotten Key to Health.* Bridgeton, Mo.: Mark A. Baker, 1989.

Cantor, Stuart. "The Diversity of Gums in Food Products." *Vegetarian Journal,* July/August 1994, p. 10–11.

Christopher, John R. *Rejuvenation through Elimination.* Springville, Ut.: Christopher Publications, 1976.

Clark, Hulda. *The Cure for All Diseases.* San Diego: Pro-Motion Publishing, 1995.

Duncan, Lindsey. "Internal Detoxification." *Healthy & Natural Journal,* Issue 1, October 1994, p. 52–55.

Flickstein, Aaron M. *Infrared Thermal System for Whole-Body Regenerative Radiant Therapy.* Glendale, Calif.: Health Mate, Inc., 1993.

Gladstar, Rosemary. "Herbal Therapeutics for the Liver." *The Science and Art of Herbology,* Lesson Two. East Barre, Vt.: Sage Publications, 1990.

Gray, Robert. *The Colon Health Handbook: New Health Through Colon Rejuvenation.* Reno: Emerald Publishing, 1991.

Gruskin, B. "Chlorophyll—Its Therapeutic Place in Acute and Supperative Disease." *American Journal of Surgery,* Vol. 19, No. 1, 1940.

Hendler, Sheldon Saul. *The Purification Prescription.* New York: William Morrow and Company, Inc., 1991.

Hoffman, David. *The Holistic Herbal.* Dorset, England: Element Books, 1983.

Jensen, Barnard. *Tissue Cleansing through Bowel Management.* Escondido, Calif.: Jensen Publications, 1981.

Kirschner, H.E. *Live Food Juices.* Monrovia, Calif.: Kirschner Publications, 1957; 39th printing, 1991.

Kloss, Jethro. *Back to Eden.* Loma Linda, Calif.: Back to Eden Books, 1988.

Kroeger, Hanna. *Parasites: The Enemy Within.* Boulder, Colo.: Hanna Kroeger, 1991.

Lust, John, *The Herb Book.* New York: Bantam Books, 1974.

Manning, Betsy Russel. *Wheatgrass Juice: Gift of Nature.* Calistoga, Calif.: Greensward Press, 1992.

Moore, Michael. *Medicinal Plants of the Pacific West.* Santa Fe: Red Crane Books, 1993.

Pizzorno, Joseph. *Total Wellness.* Rocklin, Calif.: Prima Publishing, 1996.

Reilly, Harold. *The Edgar Cayce Handbook for Health*

*through Drugless Therapy.* Virginia Beach, Va.: A.R.E. Press, 1975.

Schoeneck, Annelies. *Making Sauerkraut and Pickled Vegetables at Home.* Vancouver, B.C.: Alive Books, 1988.

Steinman, David. *Diet for a Poisoned Planet.* New York: Harmony Books, 1990.

Tierra, Michael. *The Way of Herbs.* New York: Pocket Books, 1990.

Treben, Maria. *Health through God's Pharmacy.* Steyr, Austria: Wilhelm Ennsthaler, 1988.

Ushio, Moriyasu. *The Secrets of the Ume Japanese Pickled Plum.* Magalia, Calif.: Happiness Press, 1992.

Wade, Carlson. *Inner Cleansing.* West Nyack, N.Y.: Parker Publishing, 1992.

Walker, Norman. *Colon Health: The Key to a Vibrant Life.* Prescott, Ariz.: Norwalk Press, 1979.

Walters, Richard. "Hoxsey's Herbs Heal Cancers." *Herbs and Herbal Formulas.* Taos, N.M.: Native Essence Herb Co., 1995.

Webster, David. *Acidophilus and Colon Health.* Denver: Nutri-Books, 1991.

Weil, Andrew. *Spontaneous Healing.* New York: Alfred A. Knopf, 1995.

Weinberger, Stanley. *Candida Albicans: The Quiet Epidemic.* San Anselmo, Calif.: Healing Within Products, 1995.

# *Appendix: Resources*

## Recommended books about detoxification therapies

Anderson, Richard. *Cleanse and Purify Thyself: The Clean-Me-Out Program.* Tucson, Ariz.: Richard Anderson, 1988. Available from Arise & Shine, P.O. Box 1439, Mt. Shasta, CA 96067. Well-designed herbal program, highly recommended.

Benedict, Dirk. *Confessions of a Kamikaze Cowboy.* Garden City, N.Y.: Avery Publishing Group, 1991. Memoir of actor who cured his prostate cancer with macrobiotics. Excellent description of detoxification.

Bishop, Beta. *My Triumph over Cancer.* New Canaan, Conn.: Keats Publishing, Inc., 1985. Personal experience with cancer and the Gerson therapy by a British journalist. Excellent.

Brandt, Johanna. *The Grape Cure.* Yonkers, N.Y.: Ehret Literature Publishing Company, 1932. The author toured the U.S. and other countries in the late 1920s promoting the mono-diet that cured her cancer. A classic.

Breuss, Rudolf. *The Breuss Cancer Cure.* Vancouver, B.C.: Alive Books, 1995. A famous 42-day juice fast.

Gray, Robert. *The Colon Health Handbook: New Health Through Colon Rejuvenation.* Reno: Emerald Publishing, 1991. Excellent information.

Greenfield, Louise. *Cancer Overcome by Diet: An Alternative to Surgery.* Livonia, Mich.: Midwest Publishing Company, 1987. The author cured her breast cancer with raw foods.

Jensen, Barnard. *Tissue Cleansing through Bowel Management.* Escondido, Calif.: Jensen Publications, 1981. The classic in its field; graphic photographs of expelled mucoid matter.

Mae, Eydie. *How I Conquered Breast Cancer Naturally.* Garden City Park, N.Y.: Avery Publishing Group, 1992. Best-selling memoir of breast cancer victim who studied with Ann Wigmore in the 1970s and cured herself of breast cancer with wheat grass and live foods. The author was cancer-free when she died years later in a car accident.

Native Essence Herb Company. *Herbs and Herbal Formulas.* Free brochure from Native Essence, 216M North Pueblo

#301, Taos, N.M. 87571, features well-researched articles about Essiac, Hoxsey therapy and other famous formulas.

Wigmore, Ann. *The Hippocrates Diet and Health Program.* Wayne, N.J.: Avery Publishing Group, 1984. By the woman who made wheat grass juice famous.

## Clinics

Bio-Medical Center, P.O. Box 727, 615 General Ferreira, Colonia Juarez, Tijuana, Mexico 22000, phone 011-52-6684-9011. Hoxsey therapy.

Breuss Fasting Clinic, Kurhotel Chattenbuehl, An der Rehbockswide 29 a, 34346 Hannover Muenden, Germany. Breuss juice fast.

Gerson Institute, Box 430C, Bonita, CA 91908. Gerson therapy.

Hippocrates Health Institute, 1443 Palmdale Court, West Palm Beach, FL 33411. Ann Wigmore's wheatgrass therapy.

OPAL International Health Care Center 414 Chemin Pineraie, Lac Simon Cheneville P.Q., Canada J0V 1E0. Breuss juice fast.

We Care Holistic Health Center, 1800 Long Canyon Road, Desert Hot Springs, CA. 92241.

## pH testing paper

Manufactured by Micro Essential Laboratory, Brooklyn, NY 11210, sold by Arise & Shine, P.O. Box 1439, Mt. Shasta, CA 96067; L&H Vitamins, 32-33 47th Avenue, Long Island City, NY 11101; and some health food stores.

## "Uncook" books about raw food diets

The following are only a few of the raw food books in print. Raw juices and raw fruits and vegetables are the foundation of nearly every effective detoxification program. Even if you decide not to pursue herbal detoxification, the addition of raw fruits and vegetables to your diet has important health benefits. These books offer inspiration, variety, clear instructions and appetizing recipes.

Acciardo, Marcia Madhuri. *Light Eating for Survival.* Fairfield, Ia.: 21st Century Publication, 1977. One of the best introductions to raw cuisine.

Alexander, Joe. *Blatant Raw Foodist Propaganda! or Sell Your Stove to the Junkman and Feel Great.* Nevada City, Calif.: Blue Dolphin Publishing, 1990. Entertaining, informative.

Fathman, George and Doris. *Live Foods: Nature's Perfect System of Human Nutrition.* Beaumont, Calif.: Ehret Literature Publishing Company, 1967. Personal stories, recipes.

Kenton, Leslie and Susannah. *Raw Energy.* New York: Warner Books, 1984, first published in Great Britain in 1984 by Century Publishing, Ltd. Out of print but available in some libraries or used book shops and worth the effort. Excellent research, scientific overview, good recipes.

Kulvinskas, Viktoras. *Love Your Body: Live Food Recipes.* Introduction by Dick Gregory. Fairfield, Ia.: 21st Century Publications, 1972. Written by Ann Wigmore's most prolific disciple, still popular.

Lee, William. *The Book of Raw Fruits and Vegetable Juices and Drinks.* New Canaan, Conn.: Keats Publications, Inc., 1982. One of the raw juice classics.

Walker, Norman, *The Natural Way to Vibrant Health.* Prescott, Ariz.: Norwalk Press, 1972. Author of several good handbooks.

## Herbal correspondence courses

East West Master Course in Herbology by Michael Tierra, P.O. Box 712, Santa Cruz, CA 95061.

The Science and Art of Herbalism: A Home Study Course by Rosemary Gladstar, P.O. Box 420, East Barre, VT 05649.

## Herbal organizations

American Botanical Council, P.O. Box 201660, Austin, TX 78720.

American Herb Association, P.O. Box 1673, Nevada City, CA 95959.

American Herbal Products Association, P.O. Box 4210, Austin, TX 78768.

American Herbalists Guild, P.O. Box 746555, Arvada, CA 80006-6555.

Herb Research Foundation, 1007 Pearl Street, Suite 200, Boulder, CO 80302.

International Herb Association, P.O. Box 317, Mundelein, IL 60060.

Northeast Herbal Association, P.O. Box 479, Milton, NY 12547.

## Dried herbs and teas by mail

Avena Botanicals, P.O. Box 365, West Rockport, ME 04865.

Blessed Herbs, 109 Barre Plains Road, Oakham, ME 01068.

Frontier Cooperative Herbs, P.O. Box 299, Norway, IA 52318.

Green Terrestrial, P.O. Box 41, Route 9W, Milton, NY 12547.

The Herb Closet, 104 Main Street, Montpelier, VT 05602.

HerbPharm, P.O. Box 116, Williams, OR 97544

International Herbs, Route 7 South, Bennington, VT 05201.

Island Herbs, Ryan Drum, Waldron Island, WA. 98297.

Jean's Greens, 119 Sulphur Springs Road, Newport, NY 13416.

Mountain Rose Herbs, Box 2000, Redway, CA. 95560.

Pacific Botanicals, Catalog Request, 4350 Fish Hatchery Road, Grants Pass, OR 97527.

Richters, Goodwood, Ontario LOC 1AO, Canada.

Sage Mountain Herb Products, P.O. Box 420, East Barre, VT 05649.

Trinity Herbs, P.O. Box 199, Bodega, CA 94992.

Wild Weeds, P.O. Box 88, Redway, CA 95560.

## Packaged herbal detoxification programs

Richard Anderson's Clean-Me-Out Program, Arise & Shine, P.O. Box 1439, Mt. Shasta, CA 96067. Direct mail, health food store distribution.

Robert Gray's colon health products, Holistic Horizons, P.O. Box 2868, Oakland, CA 94618. Health food store distribution.

## Clay for use in detoxification programs

Arise & Shine Hydrated Bentonite (extra thick liquid montmorillonite), Arise & Shine Herbal Products, P.O. Box 1439, Mt. Shasta, CA 96067. Mail order, health food stores.

Aztec Secret Indian Healing Clay (sun-dried green bentonite powder from Death Valley), Aztec Secret Health & Beauty, Ltd., P.O. Box 841, Pahrump, NV 89041. Health food stores.

Coso Green Clay (pure montmorillonite powder), Magick Mud, Santa Ana, CA 92704. Health food stores.

Sonne #7 (liquid bentonite montmorillonite), Sonne's Organic Foods, Inc., Kansas City, MO 64142. Health food stores.

## Nasal rinsing tools, tongue scrapers

Narial Nasal Cup, Essential Product Alliance, Inc., P.O. Box 1003, Versailles, KY 40383.

Neti Pot, Self Care, 5850 Shellmound Street, Emeryville, CA 94608-1901.

Pacific Spirit, 1334 Pacific Ave., Forest Grove, OR 97116.

## Colema boards (home colonic units)

Colema Boards of California, P.O. Box 1879, Cottonwood, CA 96022.

Ultimate Colonic Units, Ultimate Trends, Inc., 7835 South 1300 East, Sandy, UT 84094.

## Slant boards, inversion equipment

Bodylift, P.O. Box 1667, Newport Beach, CA 92663.

Pacific Spirit, 1334 Pacific Ave., Forest Grove, OR 97116.

## The five rites: recommended exercise

Kelder, Peter. *Ancient Secret of the Fountain of Youth.* Gig Harbor, Wash.: Harbor Press, 1989 reprint of 1939 handbook.

# Prebiotic foods and supplements

Schoeneck, Annelies. *Making Sauerkraut and Pickled Vegetables at Home.* Vancouver, B.C., Canada: Alive Books, 1988. (Order from Alive Books, P.O. Box 67333, Vancouver, BC, Canada V5W 3T1.)

Pressed vegetables and naturally fermented foods are rich in lactic acid, which feeds beneficial intestinal bacteria. Japanese pickle presses and ceramic German pickle crocks are available through some health food stores and mail order companies, such as Gold Mine Natural Food Company, 3419 Hancock Street, San Diego, CA. 92110-4307 and Natural Lifestyle Supply Company, 16 Lookout Drive, Asheville NC 28804.

Biotta juices, pasteurized at low temperature with added lactic acid, imported from Switzerland by Bioforce of America, Ltd., Kinderhook, NY 12106. Health food store distribution.

Jerusalem artichoke flour and tablets, rich in FOS and dietary fiber. Zumbro, Inc., 2125 Airport Drive, Faribault MN 55021. Health food store distribution.

Molkosan whey concentrate does not contain milk solids and is well-tolerated by those with milk sensitivities. Imported from Switzerland by Bioforce of America, Ltd., Kinderhook, NY 12106. Sold at a discount by mail by Willner Chemists, 100 Park Avenue, New York, NY 10017.

# Probiotic supplements

Bifidus, acidophilus and other beneficial bacteria are in plentiful supply with hundreds of products. The first reliable *Lactobacillus bifidus* product, still highly regarded, is Eugalan Forte powder, imported by BioNutritional Products, 41 Bergenline Ave., Westwood, NJ 07675 and sold by mail by L&H Vitamins, 32-33 47th Avenue, Long Island City, NY 11101. Also recommended: Jarro-Dophilus

+ FOS, sold by Willner Chemists, 100 Park Avenue, New York, NY 10017.

## Herbal Melange

Detoxifying Austrian peat, imported by La Maison Francaise #5222, Fifth Avenue, New York, NY 10185, and sold at a discount by mail by the Vitamin Shoppe, 4700 Westside Ave., North Bergen NJ 07047.

## Natur-Earth

Source of soil-based organisms (SBOs), which have significant healing properties and help prevent adverse cleansing reactions, sold by Healing Within Products, P.O. Box 1013, Larkspur, CA 94977-1013.

## Unrefined sea salt, ume plums

Eden Foods, 701 Tecumseh Road, Clinton, Mich 49236. Imports Lima Salt from France. Health food store distribution.

Grain and Salt Society, P.O. Box DD, Magalia, CA 95954. Imports Celtic Salt from France. Mail order source of salt, ume plums and miso made with unrefined salt.

Gold Mine Natural Food Company, 3419 Hancock Street, San Diego, CA 92110-4307. Mail order source of several unrefined salts, Japanese pickle presses, German pickle crocks, plus ume plums and miso made with unrefined seasalt.

# Trace mineral supplements

Concentrations vary; follow label directions, or take up to four times the recommended dose for therapeutic purposes.

T.J. Clark & Company, 1145 N. 1100 Street West, St. George, UT 84770. The T.J. Clark mine is the source of several brands of plant-derived collodial minerals.

MinerAll 72, Ameriflex, Inc., 232 NE Lincoln Street, Suite G, Hillsboro, OR 97124. A highly concentrated T.J. Clark supplement.

New Vision International, Inc. 14982 N. 83rd Place, Scottsdale, AZ 85260. Plant-derived colloidal supplement from a source other than the T.J. Clark mine.

Toxic cultural supplements

Chloramination may follow label directions or take up to ftwo tips the dose the AC-unamended rinse for it capacity purposes

1. Clark & Company, (1AS N. 110d Street West, St. Charles, MI 68770, The U.S. Clark supply the source of several brands of plant-derived cultural materials

2. MicroAB 2E Aquatiek, Inc., 229 W. Electric Street, Suite E, Hillsboro, OR 97124. A supply concentrated AC fish supplement

3. World Fisher International, Inc. 16482 W. Bath Place, Stockton, Ax 85202. Manufactural cultural supplement amendment source other than the AC fisher supplement

# INDEX